METABOLIC RESET DIET COOKBOOK FOR WOMEN OVER 50

Revitalize Your Health & Boost Metabolism with 28-Day
Rejuvenating Plan & Over 100 Tasty Recipes to Lose Weight,
Balance Hormones, Repair Liver & Reclaim Energy

Andrew H. Steve

1

About the Author

Andrew H. Steve, a renowned nutrition and health expert, specializes in empowering individuals over 40 to reclaim their health. With a passion for nutrition and a deep understanding of the human body and metabolism, Andrew has successfully guided many to achieve significant weight loss and enhanced well-being.

With over a decade of experience, Andrew's approach is far from one-size-fits-all. He tailors his advice to each individual, focusing on a holistic method that encompasses a balanced diet, mindful eating, and an active lifestyle, rather than just diets and restrictions.

Known for his ability to distill complex dietary concepts into practical, actionable strategies, Andrew is a guiding force in navigating the intricacies of metabolism and wellness. His dedication extends beyond his professional achievements, as he finds joy in outdoor activities, experimenting with new recipes, and engaging in healthy discussions.

If you're looking to lose weight, increase energy, or improve your overall well-being, Andrew H. Steve is your ideal mentor. Under his guidance, you're not just adopting a healthy lifestyle; you're embarking on a transformative journey to rediscover your vitality and thrive.

TABLE OF CONTENTS

INTRODUCTION

Understanding Metabolism

1. **Anabolism:** This is the process where the body builds molecules it needs, such as proteins and fats. It requires energy.

2. **Catabolism:** This is the process where the body breaks down molecules to obtain energy. For example, breaking down carbohydrates into glucose for energy.

Key points to comprehend about metabolism, particularly in the context of a Metabolic Reset Diet for women over 50, include:

1. Basal Metabolic Rate (BMR): BMR represents the number of calories the body needs at rest to maintain essential physiological functions, such as breathing and maintaining body temperature. Factors influencing BMR include age, gender, body composition, and genetics. Understanding one's BMR is vital for planning an effective diet and exercise routine.

2. Hormones and Metabolism: Hormones play a significant role in regulating metabolism. For women over 50, hormonal changes associated with menopause can affect metabolism. For example, a decrease in estrogen levels may lead to changes in fat distribution and a potential decrease in BMR. Understanding these hormonal shifts can help tailor the Metabolic Reset Diet to address specific needs.

3. Diet-Induced Thermogenesis: This refers to the energy expended during the digestion, absorption, and metabolism of nutrients from the food we eat. Different macronutrients (carbohydrates, proteins, and fats) have varying thermogenic effects. A Metabolic Reset Diet aims to optimize this process by focusing on nutrient-dense foods that promote efficient energy utilization.

4. Impact of Physical Activity: Regular physical activity is a key factor in maintaining a healthy metabolism. Exercise not only burns calories but also has a positive impact on muscle mass. Since muscle tissue burns more calories at rest than fat tissue, preserving or building lean muscle becomes essential, especially for women over 50.

5. Metabolic Adaptation: The body can adapt to changes in diet and exercise over time, which may affect weight loss or maintenance efforts. Understanding how the metabolism adapts can help individuals make necessary adjustments to their dietary and exercise strategies for long-term success.

Importance of a Metabolic Reset for Women Over 50

The distinct physiological changes and health considerations that come with reaching this stage of life highlight the need of a Metabolic Reset for women over 50. Hormonal fluctuations, modifications to body composition, and variations in metabolic rate become more noticeable as women approach their fifth decade and beyond.

1. **Counteracting Age-Related Metabolic Decline:**

   - With advancing age, there is a natural decline in metabolic rate, largely attributed to a reduction in muscle mass and hormonal fluctuations, particularly during menopause. This decline can result in weight gain, especially around the abdominal region, and a propensity for metabolic conditions like insulin resistance. A Metabolic Reset aims to counteract this decline, promoting efficient energy utilization and mitigating the risk of age-related metabolic issues.

2. Addressing Hormonal Changes:

- Menopause, which typically occurs in the late 40s or early 50s, brings about significant hormonal changes, including a decline in estrogen levels. This hormonal shift can impact fat distribution, increase the risk of visceral fat accumulation, and influence metabolic function. A Metabolic Reset takes into account these hormonal changes, providing a strategic approach to manage weight and optimize metabolic health during and after menopause.

3. Promoting Weight Management and Body Composition:

- Women over 50 often find it more challenging to manage their weight due to factors like a slower metabolism and changes in lifestyle. A Metabolic Reset focuses on strategies to enhance fat metabolism, preserve or build lean muscle mass, and promote a healthy body composition. This not only supports weight management but also contributes to overall well-being.

4. **Optimizing Nutrient Absorption and Utilization:**

- Age-related changes in digestive function can affect nutrient absorption. A Metabolic Reset Diet emphasizes nutrient-dense foods that are easier to digest and absorb, ensuring that the body receives essential vitamins and minerals for optimal metabolic function. This is particularly important for maintaining energy levels and supporting various physiological processes.

5. **Managing Insulin Sensitivity:**

- Insulin sensitivity tends to decrease with age, contributing to the development of conditions like type 2 diabetes. A Metabolic Reset incorporates dietary strategies to enhance insulin sensitivity, such as controlling carbohydrate intake, choosing complex carbohydrates, and incorporating regular physical activity. This proactive approach is vital for preventing and managing metabolic disorders.

6. **Improving Energy Levels and Vitality:**

- Women over 50 often experience fluctuations in energy levels, which can impact daily activities and overall vitality. A Metabolic Reset is designed to provide sustained energy through balanced nutrition and lifestyle modifications. By supporting metabolic health, individuals can experience increased energy levels, improved mood, and enhanced quality of life.

CHAPTER ONE

THE BASICS OF THE METABOLIC RESET DIET

What is the Metabolic Reset Diet?

A dietary strategy called the Metabolic Reset Diet aims to reset and improve the body's metabolism in order to support effective energy use, healthy weight management, and general wellbeing. In order to address certain metabolic needs and improve the body's capacity to burn calories efficiently, it places a strong emphasis on making deliberate modifications to eating behaviours, food intake, and meal timing.

1. **Focus on Whole, Nutrient-Dense Foods:** The diet encourages the consumption of whole, minimally processed foods rich in essential nutrients, including fruits, vegetables, lean proteins, whole grains, and healthy fats. These foods provide a wide range of vitamins, minerals, and antioxidants necessary for metabolic processes and overall health.

2. **Balanced Macronutrient Ratios:** The Metabolic Reset Diet typically promotes a balanced distribution of macronutrients—proteins, carbohydrates, and fats. Achieving the right balance helps regulate blood sugar levels, optimize energy levels, and support metabolic function. Protein intake is often emphasized to preserve or build lean muscle mass, which plays a crucial role in metabolism.

3. **Strategic Carbohydrate Intake:** The diet pays attention to the quality and quantity of carbohydrates consumed. It may involve selecting complex carbohydrates with a lower glycemic index to promote stable blood sugar levels. Controlling carbohydrate intake and timing may also be considered to manage insulin sensitivity and support metabolic health.

4. **Meal Timing and Frequency:** The Metabolic Reset Diet may incorporate principles of intermittent fasting or mindful eating to optimize meal timing. This could involve spreading meals throughout the day or implementing time-restricted eating patterns, such as fasting for a specific period and consuming meals within a designated time window. This approach aims to synchronize food intake with natural circadian rhythms and enhance metabolic efficiency.

5. **Hydration and Metabolism:** Adequate hydration is an integral part of the Metabolic Reset Diet. Water plays a vital role in various metabolic processes, including digestion and nutrient transport. Ensuring proper hydration supports overall metabolic function and can contribute to weight management.

6. **Incorporation of Metabolism-Boosting Foods:** Certain foods are believed to have metabolism-boosting properties, and the diet may include them strategically. For example, foods rich in thermogenic compounds, like certain spices and green tea, may be incorporated to enhance calorie burning. However, it's

essential to approach such aspects with a balanced and evidence-based perspective.

7. **Regular Physical Activity:** The Metabolic Reset Diet is often complemented by a focus on regular physical activity. Exercise, especially a combination of aerobic and strength training, supports muscle maintenance or growth, improves insulin sensitivity, and contributes to overall metabolic health.

8. **Adaptability and Personalization:** The Metabolic Reset Diet recognizes that individuals have unique metabolic profiles and dietary preferences. It encourages adaptability and personalization, allowing individuals to tailor the principles to their specific needs, lifestyle, and health goals.

Principles and Science Behind the Diet

The goals of the Metabolic Reset Diet are to improve general health, optimize metabolic function, and support weight management. It is based on certain scientific concepts and principles. Gaining an understanding of the fundamental ideas and scientific justifications underlying the diet might provide people important new perspectives on how and why it might work.

1. **Balancing Macronutrients:**

   - ***Principle:*** The diet emphasizes a balanced distribution of macronutrients—proteins, carbohydrates, and fats.

- ***Science:*** Each macronutrient plays a unique role in metabolism. Proteins support muscle maintenance and repair, carbohydrates provide energy, and fats are essential for hormone production and nutrient absorption. Balancing these components helps regulate blood sugar levels, manage hunger, and support overall metabolic health.

2. **Strategic Carbohydrate Management:**

   - ***Principle:*** The diet often involves strategic carbohydrate intake, focusing on the quality and quantity of carbohydrates consumed.

   - ***Science:*** Carbohydrates impact blood sugar levels, and the type and timing of carbohydrate consumption can influence insulin sensitivity. Choosing complex carbohydrates with a lower glycemic index helps maintain stable blood sugar levels, reducing the risk of insulin resistance and promoting efficient energy utilization.

3. **Intermittent Fasting or Time-Restricted Eating:**

   - ***Principle:*** The diet may incorporate principles of intermittent fasting or time-restricted eating to optimize meal timing.

   - ***Science:*** Fasting periods can enhance metabolic flexibility, encouraging the body to switch between burning glucose and fat for fuel. Time-restricted eating aligns with circadian rhythms, potentially improving metabolic efficiency and supporting weight management.

4. **Protein Emphasis for Muscle Health:**

- *Principle:* The diet often emphasizes adequate protein intake to preserve or build lean muscle mass.

- *Science:* Protein is essential for muscle maintenance and repair. As individuals age, preserving muscle mass becomes crucial for maintaining a healthy metabolism. Higher protein intake can also increase the thermic effect of food, contributing to overall energy expenditure.

5. **Hydration and Thermogenesis:**

- *Principle:* Adequate hydration is integral to the diet to support metabolic processes.

- *Science:* Water is involved in various metabolic reactions, including digestion and nutrient transport. Staying hydrated can enhance the thermic effect of food, potentially contributing to calorie burning and overall metabolic efficiency.

6. **Incorporating Metabolism-Boosting Foods:**

- *Principle:* The diet may include foods believed to boost metabolism, such as spices and certain beverages.

- *Science:* Some foods contain thermogenic compounds that can temporarily increase calorie expenditure. For example, capsaicin in chili peppers and catechins in green tea have been studied for their potential to enhance metabolic rate.

7. **Regular Physical Activity:**

   - *Principle:* The diet is often complemented by regular physical activity.

   - *Science:* Exercise has numerous metabolic benefits, including increasing energy expenditure, improving insulin sensitivity, and promoting the maintenance or growth of lean muscle mass. This synergy between diet and exercise contributes to overall metabolic health.

8. **Adaptability and Individualization:**

   - *Principle:* The diet encourages adaptability and personalization to meet individual needs and preferences.

   - *Science:* Recognizing that individuals have unique metabolic profiles, genetic factors, and dietary preferences, the diet allows for customization. This approach considers the importance of sustainability and adherence for long-term success.

Benefits for Women Over 50

For women over 50, the Metabolic Reset Diet has numerous noteworthy advantages that address the unique physiological changes and health issues that frequently coincide with this period of life. The diet offers a comprehensive strategy to improve metabolic health and general well-being, specifically designed to cater to the specific requirements of women going through menopause and aging.

1. **Weight Management and Body Composition:**

   - ***Benefit:*** The Metabolic Reset Diet helps women over 50 manage weight and optimize body composition.

   - ***Explanation:*** Age-related changes, particularly during menopause, can lead to an increased tendency for weight gain, particularly around the abdominal region. The diet, through its emphasis on balanced nutrition and muscle-preserving strategies, supports healthy weight management and encourages the maintenance or building of lean muscle mass.

2. **Improved Metabolic Rate:**

   - ***Benefit:*** The diet aims to boost and optimize the metabolic rate.

   - ***Explanation:*** As women age, there is a natural decline in metabolic rate, largely attributed to hormonal changes and a reduction in muscle mass. The Metabolic Reset Diet, with its focus on strategic macronutrient balance, protein intake, and metabolism-boosting foods, seeks to counteract this decline, promoting a more efficient metabolism.

3. **Hormonal Balance and Menopausal Symptom Relief:**

    - ***Benefit:*** The diet may contribute to hormonal balance and alleviate menopausal symptoms.

    - ***Explanation:*** Menopause brings hormonal changes, including a decline in estrogen levels. The diet's emphasis on nutrient-dense foods, particularly those rich in phytoestrogens and other beneficial compounds, may help manage hormonal fluctuations and alleviate symptoms such as hot flashes and mood swings.

4. **Enhanced Insulin Sensitivity:**

    - ***Benefit:*** The diet supports improved insulin sensitivity.

    - ***Explanation:*** Age-related changes can contribute to decreased insulin sensitivity, raising the risk of metabolic disorders like type 2 diabetes. The Metabolic Reset Diet, through its strategic carbohydrate management and emphasis on whole, nutrient-dense foods, aims to enhance insulin sensitivity and regulate blood sugar levels.

5. **Increased Energy Levels:**

    - ***Benefit:*** The diet is designed to provide sustained energy throughout the day.

- *Explanation:* Women over 50 often experience fluctuations in energy levels. The diet's focus on balanced macronutrients, nutrient-dense foods, and hydration supports stable energy levels, helping individuals maintain vitality and meet the demands of daily activities.

6. **Bone Health and Nutrient Absorption:**

   - *Benefit:* The diet promotes bone health and optimal nutrient absorption.

   - *Explanation:* Postmenopausal women are at an increased risk of osteoporosis. The diet includes foods rich in calcium, vitamin D, and other bone-supporting nutrients. Additionally, strategies to enhance nutrient absorption, such as proper hydration, contribute to overall bone health.

7. **Heart Health and Reduced Inflammation:**

   - *Benefit:* The diet supports cardiovascular health and reduces inflammation.

   - *Explanation:* Age-related changes can impact heart health, and inflammation may contribute to various health issues. The diet's focus on heart-healthy fats, antioxidants, and anti-inflammatory foods contributes to cardiovascular well-being and overall health.

8. **Promotion of Long-Term Health and Well-Being:**

- ***Benefit:*** The Metabolic Reset Diet fosters a foundation for long-term health.

- ***Explanation:*** By addressing the specific needs of women over 50 and promoting sustainable lifestyle changes, the diet supports not only immediate health goals but also lays the groundwork for continued well-being as individuals age.

BREAKFAST RECIPES

Quinoa Breakfast Bowl

Ingredients:

- 1 cup cooked quinoa
- 1/2 cup fresh berries (blueberries, strawberries)
- 1 tablespoon chia seeds
- 1 tablespoon chopped nuts (almonds, walnuts)
- 1 teaspoon honey
- 1/2 cup unsweetened almond milk

Prep Time: 10 minutes

Cooking Time: 5 minutes

Serving Time: 15 minutes

Nutritional Info: (per serving)

- Calories: 300
- Protein: 8g
- Carbohydrates: 40g
- Fat: 12g
- Fiber: 7g

Directions:

- In a bowl, combine cooked quinoa, fresh berries, chia seeds, and chopped nuts.
- Drizzle honey over the mixture and pour almond milk.

- Mix well and heat in the microwave for 1-2 minutes.
- Serve warm.

Serving Methods:

1. Serve as a warm breakfast bowl with a sprinkle of additional nuts.
2. Chill the mixture and serve as a cold quinoa parfait for a refreshing option.

Spinach and Feta Omelette

Ingredients:

- 2 eggs, beaten
- 1/2 cup fresh spinach, chopped
- 2 tablespoons feta cheese, crumbled
- 1/4 cup cherry tomatoes, sliced
- 1 teaspoon olive oil
- Salt and pepper to taste

Prep Time: 5 minutes

Cooking Time: 5 minutes

Serving Time: 10 minutes

Nutritional Info: (per serving)

- Calories: 220
- Protein: 15g
- Carbohydrates: 4g
- Fat: 16g

- Fiber: 2g

Directions:

- Heat olive oil in a non-stick pan over medium heat.
- Add chopped spinach and cook until wilted.
- Pour beaten eggs over the spinach and let it set for a moment.
- Sprinkle feta cheese and cherry tomatoes on one half of the omelette.
- Fold the omelette in half and cook until eggs are fully set.
- Season with salt and pepper.

Serving Methods:

1. Serve the omelette folded on a plate with a side of sliced avocado.
2. Roll the omelette in a whole-grain wrap for a portable breakfast option.

Greek Yogurt Parfait

Ingredients:

- 1 cup Greek yogurt
- 1/2 cup mixed berries (strawberries, raspberries)
- 2 tablespoons granola
- 1 tablespoon honey
- 1/4 teaspoon cinnamon

Prep Time: 5 minutes

Serving Time: 5 minutes

Nutritional Info: (per serving)

- Calories: 250
- Protein: 18g
- Carbohydrates: 32g
- Fat: 8g
- Fiber: 4g

Directions:

- In a glass or bowl, layer Greek yogurt, mixed berries, and granola.
- Drizzle honey over the top and sprinkle with cinnamon.
- Repeat the layers.
- Serve chilled.

Serving Methods:

1. Enjoy the parfait as a sit-down breakfast with a spoon.
2. Transfer the layers into a portable container for an on-the-go breakfast.

Sweet Potato and Kale Hash

Ingredients:

- 1 medium sweet potato, grated
- 1 cup kale, chopped
- 1/2 onion, diced
- 2 eggs
- 1 tablespoon olive oil

- Salt and pepper to taste

Prep Time: 10 minutes

Cooking Time: 10 minutes

Serving Time: 20 minutes

Nutritional Info: (per serving)

- Calories: 280
- Protein: 10g
- Carbohydrates: 28g
- Fat: 16g
- Fiber: 5g

Directions:

- Heat olive oil in a skillet over medium heat.
- Add diced onion and cook until softened.
- Add grated sweet potato and cook until slightly crispy.
- Stir in chopped kale and cook until wilted.
- Make two wells in the mixture and crack an egg into each well.
- Cover and cook until eggs are done to your liking.

Serving Methods:

1. Serve the hash on a plate with a side of sliced avocado.
2. Place the hash in a whole-grain tortilla for a breakfast burrito.

Chia Seed Pudding with Almond Butter

Ingredients:

- 2 tablespoons chia seeds
- 1/2 cup almond milk
- 1/2 teaspoon vanilla extract
- 1 tablespoon almond butter
- 1/4 cup sliced bananas
- 1 teaspoon maple syrup (optional)

Prep Time: 5 minutes

Serving Time: 3 hours (for chilling)

Nutritional Info: (per serving)

- Calories: 220
- Protein: 6g
- Carbohydrates: 17g
- Fat: 15g
- Fiber: 8g

Directions:

- In a bowl, mix chia seeds, almond milk, and vanilla extract.
- Let it sit for 5 minutes, stirring occasionally to prevent clumping.
- Transfer the mixture to a jar or glass and refrigerate for at least 3 hours or overnight.

- Top with almond butter, sliced bananas, and a drizzle of maple syrup if desired.

Serving Methods:

1. Serve the chia seed pudding in a bowl with almond butter swirled on top.
2. Layer the pudding and toppings in a glass for an aesthetically pleasing parfait.

Avocado and Smoked Salmon Toast

Ingredients:

- 1 slice whole-grain bread
- 1/2 avocado, mashed
- 2 oz smoked salmon
- 1 teaspoon capers
- Lemon wedge for garnish
- Fresh dill for garnish

Prep Time: 5 minutes

Cooking Time: 5 minutes

Serving Time: 10 minutes

Nutritional Info: (per serving)

- Calories: 280
- Protein: 15g
- Carbohydrates: 20g
- Fat: 16g

- Fiber: 7g

Directions:

- Toast the whole-grain bread slice.
- Spread mashed avocado over the toast.
- Layer smoked salmon on top.
- Garnish with capers, a squeeze of lemon juice, and fresh dill.

Serving Methods:

1. Serve the avocado and smoked salmon toast on a plate with a fork and knife.
2. Cut the toast into smaller pieces and serve as elegant appetizers for a brunch gathering.

Mango and Almond Yogurt Parfait

Ingredients:

- 1 cup Greek yogurt
- 1/2 cup diced mango
- 2 tablespoons sliced almonds
- 1 tablespoon chia seeds
- 1 teaspoon honey
- 1/4 teaspoon vanilla extract

Prep Time: 8 minutes

Serving Time: 8 minutes

Nutritional Info: (per serving)

- Calories: 290

- Protein: 18g

- Carbohydrates: 28g

- Fat: 12g

- Fiber: 4g

Directions:

- In a glass or bowl, layer Greek yogurt, diced mango, and sliced almonds.

- Sprinkle chia seeds over the layers.

- Drizzle honey and add vanilla extract.

- Repeat the layers.

- Serve chilled.

Serving Methods:

1. Enjoy the mango and almond yogurt parfait with a spoon.

2. Transfer the layers into a portable container for a nutritious breakfast on the go.

Egg White Veggie Scramble

Ingredients:

- 1 cup egg whites

- 1/2 cup cherry tomatoes, halved

- 1/4 cup bell peppers, diced

- 1/4 cup spinach, chopped

- 1 tablespoon feta cheese, crumbled

- 1 teaspoon olive oil
- Salt and pepper to taste

Prep Time: 7 minutes

Cooking Time: 5 minutes

Serving Time: 12 minutes

Nutritional Info: (per serving)

- Calories: 180
- Protein: 25g
- Carbohydrates: 8g
- Fat: 6g
- Fiber: 2g

Directions:

- Heat olive oil in a non-stick pan over medium heat.
- Add diced bell peppers and cook until slightly softened.
- Add cherry tomatoes and spinach, cooking until spinach wilts.
- Pour in egg whites and scramble until fully cooked.
- Sprinkle feta cheese over the scramble and season with salt and pepper.

Serving Methods:

1. Serve the egg white veggie scramble on a plate with a side of whole-grain toast.
2. Wrap the scramble in a whole-grain tortilla for a protein-packed breakfast burrito.

Blueberry Almond Smoothie Bowl

Ingredients:

- 1 cup frozen blueberries
- 1/2 banana
- 1/2 cup almond milk
- 1 tablespoon almond butter
- 2 tablespoons granola
- 1 tablespoon shredded coconut

Prep Time: 5 minutes

Serving Time: 5 minutes

Nutritional Info: (per serving)

- Calories: 280
- Protein: 6g
- Carbohydrates: 35g
- Fat: 14g
- Fiber: 7g

Directions:

- In a blender, combine frozen blueberries, banana, almond milk, and almond butter.
- Blend until smooth and pour into a bowl.
- Top with granola and shredded coconut.

Serving Methods:

1. Enjoy the blueberry almond smoothie bowl with a spoon.

2. Pour the smoothie into a portable cup for a nutritious and refreshing on-the-go breakfast.

Turkey and Veggie Breakfast Wrap

Ingredients:

- 1 whole-grain wrap
- 2 slices turkey breast
- 1/4 cup cherry tomatoes, sliced
- 1/4 cup cucumber, julienned
- 1 tablespoon hummus
- Fresh parsley for garnish

Prep Time: 8 minutes

Serving Time: 8 minutes

Nutritional Info: (per serving)

- Calories: 250
- Protein: 18g
- Carbohydrates: 28g
- Fat: 8g
- Fiber: 6g

Directions:

- Lay the whole-grain wrap on a flat surface.
- Spread hummus over the wrap.
- Layer turkey slices, cherry tomatoes, and julienned cucumber.
- Garnish with fresh parsley.

- Roll the wrap and slice in half.

Serving Methods:

1. Serve the turkey and veggie breakfast wrap on a plate with a side of sliced fruit.
2. Cut the wrap into bite-sized pinwheels for a delightful and shareable breakfast option.

Coconut Chia Seed Pudding

Ingredients:

- 2 tablespoons chia seeds
- 1/2 cup coconut milk
- 1/4 teaspoon vanilla extract
- 1 tablespoon shredded coconut
- 1/4 cup pineapple chunks
- 1 tablespoon sliced almonds

Prep Time: 5 minutes

Serving Time: 3 hours (for chilling)

Nutritional Info: (per serving)

- Calories: 220
- Protein: 4g
- Carbohydrates: 20g
- Fat: 15g
- Fiber: 8g

Directions:

- In a bowl, mix chia seeds, coconut milk, and vanilla extract.

- Allow it to sit for 5 minutes, stirring occasionally.

- Transfer the mixture to a jar or glass and refrigerate for at least 3 hours or overnight.

- Top with shredded coconut, pineapple chunks, and sliced almonds.

Serving Methods:

1. Serve the coconut chia seed pudding in a bowl with pineapple on the side.

2. Layer the pudding and toppings in a glass for a visually appealing parfait.

Peanut Butter Banana Smoothie

Ingredients:

- 1 ripe banana

- 2 tablespoons peanut butter

- 1 cup almond milk

- 1/2 cup Greek yogurt

- 1 tablespoon flaxseeds

- Ice cubes (optional)

Prep Time: 5 minutes

Serving Time: 5 minutes

Nutritional Info: (per serving)

- Calories: 320
- Protein: 15g
- Carbohydrates: 28g
- Fat: 18g
- Fiber: 5g

Directions:

- In a blender, combine banana, peanut butter, almond milk, Greek yogurt, and flaxseeds.
- Blend until smooth.
- Add ice cubes if desired and blend again.
- Pour into a glass and serve immediately.

Serving Methods:

1. Enjoy the peanut butter banana smoothie with a straw.
2. Pour the smoothie into a bowl and add granola and sliced banana on top.

Cauliflower and Spinach Breakfast Hash

Ingredients:

- 1 cup cauliflower rice
- 1/2 cup cherry tomatoes, halved
- 1 cup baby spinach
- 2 eggs
- 1 tablespoon olive oil
- Salt and pepper to taste

Prep Time: 7 minutes

Cooking Time: 8 minutes

Serving Time: 15 minutes

Nutritional Info: (per serving)

- Calories: 220
- Protein: 14g
- Carbohydrates: 12g
- Fat: 14g
- Fiber: 6g

Directions:

- Heat olive oil in a skillet over medium heat.
- Add cauliflower rice and cook until slightly browned.
- Stir in cherry tomatoes and baby spinach, cooking until spinach wilts.
- Create two wells in the mixture and crack an egg into each well.
- Cover and cook until eggs are done to your liking.
- Season with salt and pepper.

Serving Methods:

1. Serve the cauliflower and spinach breakfast hash on a plate with a side of sliced avocado.
2. Wrap the hash in a whole-grain tortilla for a breakfast burrito.

Berry Protein Pancakes

Ingredients:

- 1/2 cup oats, blended into flour
- 1 scoop vanilla protein powder
- 1/2 teaspoon baking powder
- 1/2 cup almond milk
- 1 egg
- 1/2 cup mixed berries (blueberries, raspberries)
- 1 tablespoon maple syrup

Prep Time: 10 minutes

Cooking Time: 10 minutes

Serving Time: 20 minutes

Nutritional Info: (per serving)

- Calories: 280
- Protein: 20g
- Carbohydrates: 35g
- Fat: 8g
- Fiber: 5g

Directions:

- In a bowl, mix oat flour, protein powder, and baking powder.
- Add almond milk and egg, stirring until well combined.
- Fold in mixed berries.

- Heat a non-stick pan over medium heat and pour batter to make pancakes.
- Cook until bubbles form on the surface, then flip and cook the other side.
- Drizzle with maple syrup before serving.

Serving Methods:

1. Serve the berry protein pancakes on a plate with a dollop of Greek yogurt.
2. Stack the pancakes and skewer with berries for a delightful breakfast kebab.

Sautéed Mushroom and Spinach Frittata

Ingredients:

- 4 eggs
- 1/2 cup mushrooms, sliced
- 1 cup baby spinach
- 1/4 cup feta cheese, crumbled
- 1 tablespoon olive oil
- Salt and pepper to taste

Prep Time: 8 minutes

Cooking Time: 12 minutes

Serving Time: 20 minutes

Nutritional Info: (per serving)

- Calories: 250

- Protein: 16g

- Carbohydrates: 4g

- Fat: 18g

- Fiber: 2g

Directions:

- Preheat the oven broiler.

- In an oven-proof skillet, heat olive oil over medium heat.

- Add sliced mushrooms and cook until softened.

- Add baby spinach and cook until wilted.

- In a bowl, beat eggs and season with salt and pepper.

- Pour the beaten eggs into the skillet, distributing evenly.

- Sprinkle crumbled feta cheese on top.

- Cook on the stovetop for 2-3 minutes, then transfer to the oven and broil until the frittata is set and slightly browned.

- Slice and serve.

Serving Methods:

1. Serve the mushroom and spinach frittata on a plate with a side of sliced tomatoes.

2. Cut the frittata into wedges and serve as an appetizer for a brunch gathering.

Protein-Packed Breakfast Burrito

Ingredients: 1 whole-grain tortilla

- 2 eggs, scrambled

- 1/4 cup black beans, drained and rinsed
- 1/4 cup diced bell peppers
- 2 tablespoons salsa
- 1 tablespoon shredded cheddar cheese
- Fresh cilantro for garnish

Prep Time: 10 minutes, ***Cooking Time:*** 5 minutes

Serving Time: 15 minutes

Nutritional Info: (per serving)

- Calories: 300
- Protein: 18g
- Carbohydrates: 30g
- Fat: 12g
- Fiber: 8g

Directions:

- Heat the whole-grain tortilla on a skillet.
- In a separate pan, scramble the eggs.
- Assemble the burrito by layering scrambled eggs, black beans, diced bell peppers, salsa, and shredded cheddar cheese.
- Garnish with fresh cilantro.
- Fold the tortilla and enjoy.

Serving Methods:

1. Serve the breakfast burrito on a plate with a side of sliced avocado.

2. Cut the burrito into bite-sized pinwheels and serve as a shareable breakfast.

Apple Cinnamon Overnight Oats

Ingredients:

- 1/2 cup rolled oats
- 1/2 cup unsweetened almond milk
- 1/2 apple, diced
- 1 tablespoon chopped walnuts
- 1/2 teaspoon cinnamon
- 1 teaspoon honey

Prep Time: 5 minutes

Serving Time: 8 hours (overnight)

Nutritional Info: (per serving)

- Calories: 240
- Protein: 6g
- Carbohydrates: 38g
- Fat: 8g
- Fiber: 7g

Directions:

- In a jar or container, combine rolled oats, almond milk, diced apple, chopped walnuts, and cinnamon.
- Stir well, cover, and refrigerate overnight.
- In the morning, drizzle honey over the oats before serving.

Serving Methods:

1. Enjoy the apple cinnamon overnight oats straight from the jar.

2. Transfer the oats to a bowl and add a dollop of Greek yogurt on top.

Turmeric and Spinach Scramble

Ingredients: 3 eggs, beaten

- 1 cup baby spinach
- 1/2 teaspoon turmeric powder
- 1/4 teaspoon cumin
- 1 tablespoon olive oil
- Salt and pepper to taste

Prep Time: 7 minutes

Cooking Time: 5 minutes

Serving Time: 12 minutes

Nutritional Info: (per serving)

- Calories: 220
- Protein: 14g
- Carbohydrates: 3g
- Fat: 18g
- Fiber: 2g

Directions: In a skillet, heat olive oil over medium heat.

- Add baby spinach and cook until wilted.

- Sprinkle turmeric and cumin over the spinach.
- Pour beaten eggs into the skillet and scramble until fully cooked.
- Season with salt and pepper.

Serving Methods:

1. Serve the turmeric and spinach scramble on a plate with a side of sliced tomatoes.
2. Roll the scramble in a whole-grain wrap for a breakfast burrito.

Mediterranean Egg Muffins

Ingredients:

- 4 eggs
- 1/4 cup feta cheese, crumbled
- 1/4 cup cherry tomatoes, diced
- 2 tablespoons black olives, sliced
- 1 tablespoon fresh basil, chopped
- Salt and pepper to taste

Prep Time: 10 minutes

Cooking Time: 15 minutes

Serving Time: 25 minutes

Nutritional Info: (per serving)

- Calories: 180
- Protein: 12g
- Carbohydrates: 4g

- Fat: 13g
- Fiber: 1g

Directions:

- Preheat the oven to 375°F (190°C).
- In a bowl, beat eggs and season with salt and pepper.
- Grease a muffin tin and distribute the egg mixture evenly.
- Top each muffin cup with feta cheese, cherry tomatoes, black olives, and fresh basil.
- Bake for 15 minutes or until the eggs are set.
- Allow to cool slightly before serving.

Serving Methods:

1. Serve the Mediterranean egg muffins on a plate with a side of mixed greens.
2. Arrange the muffins on a platter for a delightful brunch centerpiece.

Green Tea Smoothie Bowl

Ingredients:

- 1 cup brewed green tea, cooled
- 1/2 avocado
- 1/2 cup pineapple chunks
- 1 tablespoon chia seeds
- 1 tablespoon honey
- 1/4 cup granola

Prep Time: 8 minutes

Serving Time: 8 minutes

Nutritional Info: (per serving)

- Calories: 290
- Protein: 5g
- Carbohydrates: 38g
- Fat: 14g
- Fiber: 7g

Directions:

- In a blender, combine brewed green tea, avocado, pineapple chunks, and chia seeds.
- Blend until smooth.
- Pour into a bowl and top with honey and granola.

Serving Methods:

1. Enjoy the green tea smoothie bowl with a spoon.
2. Transfer the smoothie to a portable cup and sprinkle granola on top for a textured on-the-go treat.

LUNCH RECIPES

Quinoa Salad with Lemon-Tahini Dressing

Ingredients:

- 1 cup cooked quinoa
- 1 cup cherry tomatoes, halved
- 1 cucumber, diced
- 1/4 cup red onion, finely chopped
- 1/4 cup feta cheese, crumbled
- 2 tablespoons Kalamata olives, sliced
- Fresh parsley for garnish

Prep Time: 15 minutes

Cooking Time: 15 minutes (for quinoa)

Serving Time: 30 minutes

Nutritional Info: (per serving)

- Calories: 320
- Protein: 10g
- Carbohydrates: 40g
- Fat: 14g
- Fiber: 6g

Directions:

- In a large bowl, combine cooked quinoa, cherry tomatoes, cucumber, red onion, feta cheese, and olives.

- In a separate small bowl, whisk together the Lemon-Tahini Dressing ingredients.

- Pour the dressing over the salad and toss until well combined.

- Garnish with fresh parsley before serving.

Serving Methods:

1. Serve the quinoa salad on a plate with a side of grilled chicken.

2. Stuff the salad into whole-grain pita pockets for a portable lunch.

Salmon and Avocado Wrap

Ingredients:

- 1 whole-grain wrap

- 4 oz grilled salmon, flaked

- 1/2 avocado, sliced

- 1 cup mixed greens (spinach, arugula)

- 1 tablespoon Greek yogurt dill sauce

- Lemon wedges for garnish

Prep Time: 10 minutes

Cooking Time: 10 minutes (for salmon)

Serving Time: 20 minutes

Nutritional Info: (per serving)

- Calories: 340

- Protein: 25g

- Carbohydrates: 25g

- Fat: 18g
- Fiber: 8g

Directions:

- Lay the whole-grain wrap on a flat surface.
- Spread Greek yogurt dill sauce over the wrap.
- Layer grilled salmon, avocado slices, and mixed greens.
- Squeeze lemon wedges over the filling.
- Roll the wrap and slice in half.

Serving Methods:

1. Serve the salmon and avocado wrap on a plate with a side of roasted sweet potatoes.
2. Cut the wrap into bite-sized pinwheels for a delightful lunch platter.

Mushroom and Spinach Quiche

Ingredients:

- 1 pre-made whole-grain pie crust
- 4 eggs
- 1 cup mushrooms, sliced
- 1 cup baby spinach, chopped
- 1/2 cup feta cheese, crumbled
- 1 cup unsweetened almond milk
- Salt and pepper to taste

Prep Time: 20 minutes

Cooking Time: 35 minutes

Serving Time: 60 minutes

Nutritional Info: (per serving)

- Calories: 280
- Protein: 14g
- Carbohydrates: 20g
- Fat: 16g
- Fiber: 4g

Directions:

- Preheat the oven to 375°F (190°C).
- In a pan, sauté mushrooms until they release moisture.
- Add chopped spinach and cook until wilted.
- In a bowl, whisk together eggs, almond milk, salt, and pepper.
- Place the pie crust in a pie dish and add the sautéed mushrooms and spinach.
- Pour the egg mixture over the vegetables and sprinkle with crumbled feta.
- Bake for 35 minutes or until the quiche is set and slightly browned.
- Allow to cool before slicing.

Serving Methods:

1. Serve a slice of the mushroom and spinach quiche on a plate with a side of mixed greens.

2. Cut the quiche into smaller squares and serve as part of a brunch buffet.

Chickpea and Vegetable Stir-Fry

Ingredients:

- 1 cup cooked chickpeas
- 1 cup broccoli florets
- 1 bell pepper, thinly sliced
- 1 carrot, julienned
- 2 tablespoons soy sauce
- 1 tablespoon sesame oil
- 1 teaspoon ginger, minced
- 1 clove garlic, minced

Prep Time: 15 minutes

Cooking Time: 10 minutes

Serving Time: 25 minutes

Nutritional Info: (per serving)

- Calories: 280
- Protein: 12g
- Carbohydrates: 30g
- Fat: 12g
- Fiber: 8g

Directions: In a wok or skillet, heat sesame oil over medium-high heat.

- Add minced ginger and garlic, stirring for 1 minute.

- Add broccoli, bell pepper, and julienned carrot, stir-frying until vegetables are tender-crisp.
- Stir in cooked chickpeas.
- Pour soy sauce over the stir-fry and toss until well-coated.
- Serve immediately.

Serving Methods:

1. Serve the chickpea and vegetable stir-fry on a bed of quinoa.
2. Wrap the stir-fry in large lettuce leaves for a low-carb option.

Turkey and Quinoa Stuffed Peppers

Ingredients:

- 4 bell peppers, halved and seeds removed
- 1 cup cooked quinoa
- 1/2 lb ground turkey
- 1 cup black beans, drained and rinsed
- 1 cup corn kernels
- 1 teaspoon chili powder
- 1/2 teaspoon cumin
- 1/4 cup shredded cheddar cheese
- Fresh cilantro for garnish

Prep Time: 20 minutes

Cooking Time: 30 minutes

Serving Time: 50 minutes

Nutritional Info: (per serving)

- Calories: 320

- Protein: 22g

- Carbohydrates: 30g

- Fat: 14g

- Fiber: 8g

Directions:

- Preheat the oven to 375°F (190°C).

- In a skillet, brown ground turkey over medium heat.

- Stir in cooked quinoa, black beans, corn, chili powder, and cumin.

- Spoon the mixture into halved bell peppers.

- Sprinkle shredded cheddar cheese on top.

- Bake for 30 minutes or until peppers are tender.

- Garnish with fresh cilantro before serving.

Serving Methods:

1. Serve the turkey and quinoa stuffed peppers on a plate with a side of Greek salad.

2. Arrange the stuffed peppers on a platter for a colorful and filling lunch spread.

Caprese Chicken Salad

Ingredients:

- 2 boneless, skinless chicken breasts, grilled and sliced

- 1 cup cherry tomatoes, halved

- 1 cup fresh mozzarella balls
- Fresh basil leaves for garnish
- Balsamic glaze for drizzling
- Salt and pepper to taste

Prep Time: 15 minutes

Cooking Time: 15 minutes (for grilling chicken)

Serving Time: 30 minutes

Nutritional Info: (per serving)

- Calories: 320
- Protein: 30g
- Carbohydrates: 5g
- Fat: 18g
- Fiber: 1g

Directions:

- In a bowl, combine sliced grilled chicken, cherry tomatoes, and fresh mozzarella.
- Season with salt and pepper.
- Arrange the mixture on a plate and garnish with fresh basil leaves.
- Drizzle with balsamic glaze before serving.

Serving Methods:

1. Serve the Caprese chicken salad alongside a whole-grain roll.

2. Assemble the salad in a mason jar for a convenient and portable lunch option.

Lentil and Vegetable Soup

Ingredients:

- 1 cup dried lentils, rinsed and drained
- 1 onion, diced
- 2 carrots, chopped
- 2 celery stalks, chopped
- 3 cloves garlic, minced
- 1 can (14 oz) diced tomatoes
- 6 cups vegetable broth
- 1 teaspoon cumin
- 1/2 teaspoon smoked paprika
- Salt and pepper to taste

Prep Time: 15 minutes

Cooking Time: 30 minutes

Serving Time: 45 minutes

Nutritional Info: (per serving)

- Calories: 280
- Protein: 16g
- Carbohydrates: 45g
- Fat: 2g
- Fiber: 18g

Directions:

- In a large pot, sauté onion, carrots, and celery until softened.
- Add minced garlic, cumin, and smoked paprika, stirring for 1 minute.
- Pour in lentils, diced tomatoes, and vegetable broth.
- Bring to a boil, then reduce heat and simmer until lentils are tender.
- Season with salt and pepper before serving.

Serving Methods:

1. Serve the lentil and vegetable soup in a bowl with a side of whole-grain crackers.
2. Pour the soup into a thermos for a warm and hearty lunch on the go.

Grilled Shrimp and Quinoa Bowl

Ingredients: 8 oz shrimp, peeled and deveined

- 1 cup cooked quinoa
- 1 cup broccoli florets
- 1 bell pepper, sliced
- 1 tablespoon olive oil
- 1 teaspoon lemon zest
- Fresh parsley for garnish

Prep Time: 20 minutes

Cooking Time: 10 minutes (for shrimp)

Serving Time: 30 minutes

Nutritional Info: (per serving)

- Calories: 290
- Protein: 25g
- Carbohydrates: 25g
- Fat: 10g
- Fiber: 5g

Directions:

- Toss shrimp, broccoli, and bell pepper in olive oil and lemon zest.
- Grill shrimp until cooked through and vegetables are slightly charred.
- In a bowl, layer cooked quinoa, grilled shrimp, and vegetables.
- Garnish with fresh parsley before serving.

Serving Methods:

1. Serve the grilled shrimp and quinoa bowl on a plate with a side of mixed greens.
2. Pack the bowl in a lunch container with a separate dressing for a portable meal.

Eggplant and Chickpea Salad

Ingredients: 1 large eggplant, cubed

- 1 can (15 oz) chickpeas, drained and rinsed
- 1 red onion, thinly sliced

- 1/4 cup fresh mint, chopped
- 1/4 cup feta cheese, crumbled
- 2 tablespoons balsamic vinegar
- 2 tablespoons olive oil
- Salt and pepper to taste

Prep Time: 20 minutes

Cooking Time: 15 minutes (for roasting eggplant)

Serving Time: 35 minutes

Nutritional Info: (per serving)

- Calories: 250
- Protein: 10g
- Carbohydrates: 30g
- Fat: 10g
- Fiber: 8g

Directions: Preheat the oven to 400°F (200°C).

- Toss eggplant cubes in olive oil, salt, and pepper, then roast until golden brown.
- In a bowl, combine roasted eggplant, chickpeas, red onion, mint, and feta.
- Drizzle with balsamic vinegar before serving.

Serving Methods:

1. Serve the eggplant and chickpea salad on a plate with a side of whole-grain bread.

2. Layer the salad in a mason jar for a visually appealing and portable lunch.

Turkey and Vegetable Stir-Fry

Ingredients: 1 lb turkey breast, thinly sliced

- 2 cups broccoli florets
- 1 bell pepper, sliced
- 1 zucchini, sliced
- 2 tablespoons low-sodium soy sauce
- 1 tablespoon hoisin sauce
- 1 tablespoon sesame oil
- 1 teaspoon ginger, minced

Prep Time: 15 minutes

Cooking Time: 10 minutes

Serving Time: 25 minutes

Nutritional Info: (per serving)

- Calories: 280
- Protein: 30g
- Carbohydrates: 15g
- Fat: 10g
- Fiber: 5g

Directions: In a wok or skillet, heat sesame oil over medium-high heat.

- Add sliced turkey and cook until browned.

- Stir in broccoli, bell pepper, zucchini, and minced ginger.
- Mix in soy sauce and hoisin sauce, ensuring everything is well-coated.
- Serve immediately.

Serving Methods:

1. Serve the turkey and vegetable stir-fry on a bed of cauliflower rice.
2. Wrap the stir-fry in large lettuce leaves for a low-carb lunch option.

Mediterranean Quinoa Bowl

Ingredients:

- 1 cup cooked quinoa
- 1/2 cup cherry tomatoes, halved
- 1/4 cup cucumber, diced
- 1/4 cup Kalamata olives, sliced
- 1/4 cup feta cheese, crumbled
- 2 tablespoons extra-virgin olive oil
- Fresh oregano for garnish

Prep Time: 15 minutes

Serving Time: 15 minutes

Nutritional Info: (per serving)

- Calories: 280
- Protein: 10g

- Carbohydrates: 30g

- Fat: 14g

- Fiber: 6g

Directions:

- In a bowl, combine cooked quinoa, cherry tomatoes, cucumber, olives, and feta cheese.

- Drizzle with extra-virgin olive oil and toss until well-coated.

- Garnish with fresh oregano before serving.

Serving Methods:

1. Serve the Mediterranean quinoa bowl on a plate with a side of grilled lemon herb chicken.

2. Pack the quinoa bowl in a bento-style lunchbox for a portable and vibrant lunch.

Vegetarian Black Bean Quesadillas

Ingredients: 4 whole-grain tortillas

- 1 can (15 oz) black beans, mashed

- 1 cup corn kernels

- 1 cup bell peppers, diced

- 1 cup shredded Monterey Jack cheese

- 1 tablespoon olive oil

- Salsa and guacamole for serving

Prep Time: 20 minutes

Cooking Time: 10 minutes

Serving Time: 30 minutes

Nutritional Info: (per serving)

- Calories: 320
- Protein: 15g
- Carbohydrates: 40g
- Fat: 12g
- Fiber: 8g

Directions:

- In a skillet, heat olive oil over medium heat.
- Place one tortilla in the skillet, spread mashed black beans, corn, bell peppers, and cheese.
- Top with another tortilla and cook until golden brown on both sides.
- Repeat for the remaining quesadillas.
- Slice into wedges and serve with salsa and guacamole.

Serving Methods:

1. Serve the vegetarian black bean quesadillas on a plate with a side of mixed greens.
2. Cut into smaller triangles and serve as a shareable appetizer for lunch gatherings.

Asian-Inspired Salmon Bowl

Ingredients: 1 cup cooked brown rice

- 8 oz grilled salmon, flaked

- 1 cup broccoli florets, steamed

- 1 carrot, julienned

- 2 tablespoons low-sodium soy sauce

- 1 tablespoon rice vinegar

- 1 teaspoon sesame oil

- Sesame seeds for garnish

Prep Time: 20 minutes

Cooking Time: 15 minutes (for salmon)

Serving Time: 35 minutes

Nutritional Info: (per serving)

- Calories: 340, Protein: 25g

- Carbohydrates: 30g

- Fat: 14g

- Fiber: 6g

Directions: In a bowl, assemble cooked brown rice, grilled salmon, steamed broccoli, and julienned carrots.

- In a small bowl, whisk together soy sauce, rice vinegar, and sesame oil.

- Drizzle the sauce over the bowl and toss gently.

- Garnish with sesame seeds before serving.

Serving Methods:

1. Serve the Asian-inspired salmon bowl on a plate with a side of pickled ginger.

2. Pack the bowl in a segmented lunch container for a balanced and flavorful meal.

Spaghetti Squash Primavera

Ingredients: 1 medium spaghetti squash, cooked and shredded

- 1 cup cherry tomatoes, halved
- 1 cup zucchini, sliced
- 1 cup bell peppers, julienned
- 2 cloves garlic, minced
- 2 tablespoons olive oil
- Fresh basil for garnish
- Grated Parmesan cheese (optional)

Prep Time: 20 minutes

Cooking Time: 30 minutes (for squash)

Serving Time: 50 minutes

Nutritional Info: (per serving)

- Calories: 250
- Protein: 5g
- Carbohydrates: 30g
- Fat: 14g
- Fiber: 8g

Directions: In a skillet, sauté garlic in olive oil until fragrant.

- Add cherry tomatoes, zucchini, and bell peppers, cooking until vegetables are tender.

- Toss in shredded spaghetti squash and mix well.

- Garnish with fresh basil and Parmesan cheese if desired.

Serving Methods:

1. Serve the spaghetti squash primavera on a plate with a sprinkle of pine nuts.

2. Portion the dish into individual containers for an easy and reheatable lunch.

Chicken and Vegetable Lettuce Wraps

Ingredients:

- 1 lb ground chicken

- 1 cup cabbage, shredded

- 1 carrot, grated

- 1/4 cup hoisin sauce

- 2 tablespoons soy sauce

- 1 tablespoon sesame oil

- Butter lettuce leaves for wrapping

- Green onions for garnish

Prep Time: 15 minutes

Cooking Time: 15 minutes

Serving Time: 30 minutes

Nutritional Info: (per serving)

- Calories: 290

- Protein: 20g

- Carbohydrates: 15g

- Fat: 18g

- Fiber: 5g

Directions:

- In a skillet, brown ground chicken over medium heat.

- Add shredded cabbage and grated carrot, cooking until vegetables are softened.

- In a small bowl, mix hoisin sauce, soy sauce, and sesame oil.

- Pour the sauce over the chicken mixture and stir to combine.

- Spoon the chicken mixture into lettuce leaves and garnish with green onions.

Serving Methods:

1. Serve the chicken and vegetable lettuce wraps on a plate with a side of sliced cucumber.

2. Arrange the wraps on a platter for a fun and interactive lunch experience.

Sweet Potato and Chickpea Buddha Bowl

Ingredients:

- 1 cup roasted sweet potatoes, cubed

- 1 cup cooked chickpeas

- 1 cup kale, massaged

- 1/2 avocado, sliced

- 2 tablespoons tahini dressing

- Pumpkin seeds for garnish

Prep Time: 20 minutes

Cooking Time: 30 minutes (for sweet potatoes)

Serving Time: 50 minutes

Nutritional Info: (per serving)

- Calories: 320
- Protein: 12g
- Carbohydrates: 35g
- Fat: 15g
- Fiber: 10g

Directions:

- Assemble roasted sweet potatoes, chickpeas, massaged kale, and avocado in a bowl.
- Drizzle with tahini dressing and toss gently.
- Garnish with pumpkin seeds before serving.

Serving Methods:

1. Serve the sweet potato and chickpea Buddha bowl on a plate with a side of quinoa.
2. Pack the bowl in a divided lunch container for a well-balanced and visually appealing meal.

Turkey and Cranberry Wrap

Ingredients: 1 whole-grain wrap

- 4 oz sliced turkey breast
- 2 tablespoons cranberry sauce
- 1/4 cup baby spinach
- 1 tablespoon cream cheese
- Pecans for crunch

Prep Time: 10 minutes

Serving Time: 10 minutes

Nutritional Info: (per serving)

- Calories: 280
- Protein: 20g
- Carbohydrates: 25g
- Fat: 12g
- Fiber: 4g

Directions:

- Lay the whole-grain wrap on a flat surface.
- Spread cream cheese on the wrap.
- Layer sliced turkey, cranberry sauce, baby spinach, and pecans.
- Roll the wrap and slice in half.

Serving Methods:

1. Serve the turkey and cranberry wrap on a plate with a side of mixed berries.

2. Cut the wrap into bite-sized pinwheels for a festive and shareable lunch.

Quinoa and Black Bean Stuffed Bell Peppers

Ingredients:

- 4 bell peppers, halved and seeds removed
- 1 cup cooked quinoa
- 1 can (15 oz) black beans, drained and rinsed
- 1 cup corn kernels
- 1 cup salsa
- 1 teaspoon cumin
- 1/2 teaspoon chili powder
- 1/4 cup shredded pepper jack cheese
- Fresh cilantro for garnish

Prep Time: 20 minutes

Cooking Time: 30 minutes

Serving Time: 50 minutes

Nutritional Info: (per serving)

- Calories: 310
- Protein: 15g
- Carbohydrates: 50g
- Fat: 5g
- Fiber: 10g

Directions: Preheat the oven to 375°F (190°C).

- In a bowl, combine cooked quinoa, black beans, corn, salsa, cumin, and chili powder.
- Stuff the bell pepper halves with the quinoa mixture.
- Top with shredded pepper jack cheese.
- Bake for 30 minutes or until peppers are tender.
- Garnish with fresh cilantro before serving.

Serving Methods:

1. Serve the quinoa and black bean stuffed bell peppers on a plate with a side of guacamole.
2. Arrange the stuffed peppers on a platter for a colorful and nutritious lunch presentation.

Zucchini Noodles with Pesto and Cherry Tomatoes

Ingredients:

- 2 zucchinis, spiralized
- 1 cup cherry tomatoes, halved
- 1/4 cup pine nuts, toasted
- 1/4 cup fresh basil pesto
- Parmesan cheese for garnish
- Lemon wedges for serving

Prep Time: 15 minutes

Serving Time: 15 minutes

Nutritional Info: (per serving)

- Calories: 250

- Protein: 8g

- Carbohydrates: 12g

- Fat: 20g

- Fiber: 4g

Directions:

- Spiralize zucchinis into noodle-like strands.

- In a pan, sauté zucchini noodles until slightly softened.

- Toss in cherry tomatoes, toasted pine nuts, and fresh basil pesto.

- Garnish with Parmesan cheese and serve with lemon wedges.

Serving Methods:

1. Serve the zucchini noodles with pesto on a plate with a side of grilled shrimp.

2. Pack the dish in a glass container for a refreshing and light lunch.

Cauliflower and Chickpea Curry

Ingredients:

- 1 cup cauliflower florets

- 1 can (15 oz) chickpeas, drained and rinsed

- 1 cup spinach leaves

- 1 onion, finely chopped

- 2 cloves garlic, minced

- 1 tablespoon curry powder

- 1 teaspoon turmeric

- 1 can (14 oz) coconut milk

- Fresh cilantro for garnish

- Brown rice for serving

Prep Time: 20 minutes

Cooking Time: 25 minutes

Serving Time: 45 minutes

Nutritional Info: (per serving)

- Calories: 280

- Protein: 10g

- Carbohydrates: 35g

- Fat: 12g

- Fiber: 8g

Directions: In a pan, sauté chopped onion and minced garlic until translucent.

- Add cauliflower florets, chickpeas, curry powder, and turmeric, stirring to coat.

- Pour in coconut milk and simmer until cauliflower is tender.

- Fold in spinach leaves and cook until wilted.

- Garnish with fresh cilantro and serve over brown rice.

Serving Methods:

1. Serve the cauliflower and chickpea curry on a plate with a side of naan bread.

2. Spoon the curry into individual containers for a flavorful and reheatable lunch.

DINNER RECIPES

Salmon and Asparagus Foil Packets

Ingredients:

- 4 salmon fillets
- 1 bunch asparagus, trimmed
- 2 tablespoons olive oil
- 1 lemon, sliced
- Fresh dill for garnish
- Salt and pepper to taste

Prep Time: 15 minutes

Cooking Time: 20 minutes

Serving Time: 35 minutes

Nutritional Info: (per serving)

- Calories: 320
- Protein: 30g
- Carbohydrates: 8g
- Fat: 20g
- Fiber: 4g

Directions:

- Preheat the oven to 400°F (200°C).
- Place each salmon fillet on a piece of foil.
- Arrange asparagus around the salmon.

- Drizzle with olive oil, season with salt and pepper, and top with lemon slices.

- Seal the foil packets and bake for 20 minutes.

- Garnish with fresh dill before serving.

Serving Methods:

1. Serve the salmon and asparagus foil packets on a plate with a side of quinoa.

2. Unwrap the packets and transfer the contents to a bowl for a rustic and communal dinner.

Vegetarian Stir-Fried Cauliflower Rice

Ingredients:

- 1 head cauliflower, grated

- 1 cup mixed vegetables (bell peppers, peas, carrots)

- 2 eggs, beaten

- 3 tablespoons soy sauce

- 1 tablespoon sesame oil

- 2 green onions, sliced

- Sesame seeds for garnish

Prep Time: 15 minutes

Cooking Time: 15 minutes

Serving Time: 30 minutes

Nutritional Info: (per serving)

- Calories: 220

- Protein: 10g
- Carbohydrates: 25g
- Fat: 10g
- Fiber: 8g

Directions:

- In a wok or skillet, heat sesame oil over medium-high heat.
- Add grated cauliflower and stir-fry for 5 minutes.
- Push cauliflower to one side and scramble eggs on the other side.
- Mix in mixed vegetables and soy sauce, stir-frying until veggies are tender.
- Garnish with sliced green onions and sesame seeds before serving.

Serving Methods:

1. Serve the stir-fried cauliflower rice on a plate with a side of tofu skewers.
2. Create lettuce wraps by spooning the mixture into large lettuce leaves for a low-carb option.

Grilled Chicken and Vegetable Skewers

Ingredients: 1 lb chicken breast, cubed

- 1 zucchini, sliced
- 1 red onion, diced
- 1 bell pepper, cut into chunks

- 2 tablespoons olive oil

- 1 teaspoon Italian seasoning

- Salt and pepper to taste

Prep Time: 20 minutes

Cooking Time: 15 minutes

Serving Time: 35 minutes

Nutritional Info: (per serving)

- Calories: 280

- Protein: 30g

- Carbohydrates: 10g

- Fat: 12g

- Fiber: 3g

Directions: Preheat the grill to medium-high heat.

- Thread chicken, zucchini, red onion, and bell pepper onto skewers.

- Brush with olive oil and sprinkle with Italian seasoning, salt, and pepper.

- Grill for 15 minutes, turning occasionally until chicken is cooked through.

- Serve the skewers on a plate.

Serving Methods:

1. Serve the grilled chicken and vegetable skewers with a side of quinoa.

2. Slide the ingredients off the skewers and onto a bed of mixed greens for a refreshing salad.

Shrimp and Broccoli Stir-Fry

Ingredients:

- 8 oz shrimp, peeled and deveined
- 2 cups broccoli florets
- 1 bell pepper, sliced
- 2 tablespoons low-sodium soy sauce
- 1 tablespoon honey
- 1 tablespoon ginger, minced
- 1 clove garlic, minced

Prep Time: 15 minutes

Cooking Time: 10 minutes

Serving Time: 25 minutes

Nutritional Info: (per serving)

- Calories: 250
- Protein: 25g
- Carbohydrates: 20g
- Fat: 8g
- Fiber: 4g

Directions:

- In a wok or skillet, heat oil over medium-high heat.
- Add shrimp and cook until pink.

- Add broccoli and bell pepper, stir-frying until vegetables are crisp-tender.
- In a small bowl, mix soy sauce, honey, ginger, and garlic.
- Pour the sauce over the shrimp and vegetables, tossing to coat.
- Serve immediately.

Serving Methods:

1. Serve the shrimp and broccoli stir-fry over brown rice.
2. Wrap the stir-fry in whole-grain tortillas for a quick and portable dinner.

Mushroom and Spinach Stuffed Chicken Breast

Ingredients:

- 4 boneless, skinless chicken breasts
- 1 cup mushrooms, finely chopped
- 2 cups baby spinach
- 1/4 cup feta cheese, crumbled
- 1 tablespoon olive oil
- 1 teaspoon garlic powder
- Salt and pepper to taste

Prep Time: 25 minutes

Cooking Time: 25 minutes

Serving Time: 50 minutes

Nutritional Info: (per serving)

- Calories: 320

- Protein: 30g

- Carbohydrates: 5g

- Fat: 18g

- Fiber: 2g

Directions:

- Preheat the oven to 375°F (190°C).

- In a skillet, sauté mushrooms and spinach in olive oil until wilted.

- Butterfly each chicken breast and stuff with the mushroom-spinach mixture and crumbled feta.

- Season the outside of the chicken with garlic powder, salt, and pepper.

- Bake for 25 minutes or until the chicken is cooked through.

- Serve the stuffed chicken breasts on a plate.

Serving Methods:

1. Serve the mushroom and spinach stuffed chicken breasts with a side of roasted sweet potatoes.

2. Slice the stuffed chicken and arrange on a platter for an elegant dinner presentation.

Turkey and Vegetable Quinoa Bowl

Ingredients:

- 1 cup cooked quinoa

- 1 lb ground turkey

- 1 zucchini, diced

- 1 bell pepper, chopped

- 1 cup cherry tomatoes, halved

- 2 tablespoons olive oil

- 1 teaspoon cumin

- 1/2 teaspoon smoked paprika

- Salt and pepper to taste

Prep Time: 20 minutes

Cooking Time: 20 minutes

Serving Time: 40 minutes

Nutritional Info: (per serving)

- Calories: 310

- Protein: 25g

- Carbohydrates: 30g

- Fat: 12g

- Fiber: 5g

Directions:

- In a skillet, heat olive oil over medium heat.

- Brown ground turkey until cooked through.

- Add diced zucchini, bell pepper, and cherry tomatoes.

- Season with cumin, smoked paprika, salt, and pepper.

- Stir in cooked quinoa and mix until well combined.

- Serve the turkey and vegetable quinoa bowl on a plate.

Serving Methods:

1. Garnish the bowl with fresh cilantro and a squeeze of lime juice for added freshness.

2. Portion the mixture into bell pepper halves and bake for a creative and colorful presentation.

Lemon Herb Baked Cod

Ingredients:

- 4 cod fillets
- 2 tablespoons olive oil
- 1 lemon, juiced and zested
- 2 cloves garlic, minced
- 1 tablespoon fresh parsley, chopped
- Salt and pepper to taste

Prep Time: 15 minutes

Cooking Time: 20 minutes

Serving Time: 35 minutes

Nutritional Info: (per serving)

- Calories: 180
- Protein: 25g
- Carbohydrates: 2g
- Fat: 8g
- Fiber: 0g

Directions: Preheat the oven to 400°F (200°C).

- Place cod fillets on a baking sheet.

- In a bowl, mix olive oil, lemon juice, lemon zest, minced garlic, salt, and pepper.

- Pour the mixture over the cod fillets.

- Bake for 20 minutes or until the fish flakes easily.

- Garnish with fresh parsley and serve on a plate.

Serving Methods:

1. Pair the lemon herb baked cod with a side of steamed asparagus for a complete meal.

2. Serve over a bed of sautéed spinach for a light and vibrant dinner.

Chickpea and Vegetable Curry

Ingredients:

- 1 can (15 oz) chickpeas, drained and rinsed

- 1 cup cauliflower florets

- 1 cup sweet potatoes, diced

- 1 cup cherry tomatoes, halved

- 1 onion, finely chopped

- 2 tablespoons curry powder

- 1 can (14 oz) coconut milk

- Fresh cilantro for garnish

Prep Time: 25 minutes

Cooking Time: 30 minutes

Serving Time: 55 minutes

Nutritional Info: (per serving)

- Calories: 280
- Protein: 8g
- Carbohydrates: 35g
- Fat: 12g
- Fiber: 10g

Directions:

- In a pot, sauté chopped onion until translucent.
- Add curry powder and stir for 1 minute.
- Add chickpeas, cauliflower, sweet potatoes, cherry tomatoes, and coconut milk.
- Simmer until vegetables are tender.
- Garnish with fresh cilantro and serve in a bowl.

Serving Methods:

1. Serve the chickpea and vegetable curry over brown rice for a hearty dinner.
2. Spoon the curry into individual serving bowls with a side of naan bread for dipping.

Quinoa Stuffed Bell Peppers

Ingredients:

- 4 bell peppers, halved and seeds removed
- 1 cup cooked quinoa

- 1 lb ground chicken
- 1 cup black beans, drained and rinsed
- 1 cup corn kernels
- 1 teaspoon cumin
- 1/2 teaspoon chili powder
- 1/4 cup shredded cheddar cheese
- Fresh cilantro for garnish

Prep Time: 30 minutes

Cooking Time: 30 minutes

Serving Time: 60 minutes

Nutritional Info: (per serving)

- Calories: 320
- Protein: 25g
- Carbohydrates: 30g
- Fat: 12g
- Fiber: 6g

Directions:

- Preheat the oven to 375°F (190°C).
- In a skillet, brown ground chicken.
- In a bowl, mix cooked quinoa, black beans, corn, cumin, and chili powder.
- Stuff the bell pepper halves with the quinoa mixture.
- Top with shredded cheddar cheese.

- Bake for 30 minutes or until peppers are tender.
- Garnish with fresh cilantro and serve on a plate.

Serving Methods:

1. Serve the quinoa stuffed bell peppers with a side of guacamole for added creaminess.
2. Create a colorful dinner plate by adding a variety of roasted vegetables on the side.

Mushroom and Lentil Soup

Ingredients:

- 1 cup brown lentils, rinsed and drained
- 1 onion, diced
- 2 carrots, chopped
- 2 celery stalks, sliced
- 8 oz mushrooms, sliced
- 3 cloves garlic, minced
- 1 can (14 oz) diced tomatoes
- 8 cups vegetable broth
- 1 teaspoon thyme
- Salt and pepper to taste

Prep Time: 20 minutes

Cooking Time: 40 minutes

Serving Time: 60 minutes

Nutritional Info: (per serving)

- Calories: 250
- Protein: 15g
- Carbohydrates: 40g
- Fat: 2g
- Fiber: 18g

Directions:

- In a large pot, sauté onion, carrots, celery, and mushrooms until softened.
- Add minced garlic and cook for 1 minute.
- Pour in lentils, diced tomatoes, vegetable broth, thyme, salt, and pepper.
- Bring to a boil, then reduce heat and simmer until lentils are tender.
- Adjust seasoning and serve the mushroom and lentil soup in a bowl.

Serving Methods:

1. Serve the soup with a side of whole-grain bread for a comforting dinner.
2. Pour the soup into a thermos for a warm and nourishing meal on the go.

Sweet Potato and Kale Stuffed Portobello Mushrooms

Ingredients: 4 large portobello mushrooms, stems removed

- 2 cups sweet potatoes, cubed
- 2 cups kale, chopped

- 1 onion, diced
- 2 cloves garlic, minced
- 2 tablespoons olive oil
- 1/4 cup Parmesan cheese, grated
- Salt and pepper to taste

Prep Time: 25 minutes

Cooking Time: 30 minutes

Serving Time: 55 minutes

Nutritional Info: (per serving)

- Calories: 280
- Protein: 8g
- Carbohydrates: 40g
- Fat: 10g
- Fiber: 8g

Directions: Preheat the oven to 375°F (190°C).

- Place portobello mushrooms on a baking sheet.
- In a skillet, sauté onions and garlic in olive oil until softened.
- Add sweet potatoes and kale, cooking until vegetables are tender.
- Season with salt and pepper, then spoon the mixture into the mushrooms.
- Sprinkle Parmesan cheese on top.
- Bake for 20-25 minutes or until mushrooms are cooked through.
- Serve the stuffed portobello mushrooms on a plate.

Serving Methods:

1. Garnish with fresh thyme and serve alongside a quinoa pilaf for a well-rounded meal.

2. Pair with a side of mixed greens dressed with balsamic vinaigrette for a light and refreshing dinner.

Spiced Lentil and Vegetable Stew

Ingredients:

- 1 cup dry green or brown lentils, rinsed
- 1 onion, diced
- 2 carrots, sliced
- 2 celery stalks, chopped
- 1 bell pepper, diced
- 3 cloves garlic, minced
- 1 can (14 oz) crushed tomatoes
- 6 cups vegetable broth
- 1 teaspoon cumin
- 1/2 teaspoon smoked paprika
- 1/4 teaspoon cayenne pepper
- Fresh parsley for garnish

Prep Time: 20 minutes

Cooking Time: 40 minutes

Serving Time: 60 minutes

Nutritional Info: (per serving)

- Calories: 240
- Protein: 15g
- Carbohydrates: 40g
- Fat: 2g
- Fiber: 16g

Directions:

- In a large pot, sauté onions, carrots, celery, and bell pepper until softened.

- Add minced garlic, cumin, smoked paprika, and cayenne pepper. Stir for 1 minute.
- Pour in lentils, crushed tomatoes, and vegetable broth.
- Bring to a boil, then reduce heat and simmer until lentils are tender.
- Adjust seasoning and serve the spiced lentil and vegetable stew in a bowl.

Serving Methods:

1. Top the stew with a dollop of Greek yogurt and a sprinkle of pumpkin seeds for added creaminess and crunch.
2. Serve over a bed of quinoa or brown rice for a satisfying and complete dinner.

Baked Eggplant Parmesan

Ingredients:

- 2 large eggplants, sliced
- 2 cups marinara sauce
- 1 cup whole-wheat breadcrumbs
- 1 cup mozzarella cheese, shredded
- 1/2 cup Parmesan cheese, grated
- Fresh basil for garnish
- Salt and pepper to taste

Prep Time: 30 minutes

Cooking Time: 30 minutes

Serving Time: 60 minutes

Nutritional Info: (per serving)

- Calories: 280
- Protein: 12g
- Carbohydrates: 35g

- Fat: 10g
- Fiber: 12g

Directions:

- Preheat the oven to 400°F (200°C).
- Lay eggplant slices on a baking sheet and sprinkle with salt. Let sit for 15 minutes, then pat dry.
- Dip each slice in marinara sauce, then coat with breadcrumbs.
- Arrange the slices in a baking dish, layering with marinara sauce and mozzarella cheese.
- Repeat the layers and top with Parmesan cheese.
- Bake for 25-30 minutes or until golden and bubbly.
- Garnish with fresh basil and serve on a plate.

Serving Methods:

1. Serve the baked eggplant Parmesan with a side of whole-grain spaghetti.
2. Layer the slices between whole-grain bread for a delicious eggplant Parmesan sandwich.

Teriyaki Tofu Stir-Fry

Ingredients:

- 1 lb firm tofu, cubed
- 2 cups broccoli florets
- 1 red bell pepper, sliced
- 1 carrot, julienned
- 2 tablespoons low-sodium teriyaki sauce
- 1 tablespoon sesame oil
- 1 tablespoon rice vinegar
- Sesame seeds for garnish

Prep Time: 25 minutes

Cooking Time: 20 minutes

Serving Time: 45 minutes

Nutritional Info: (per serving)

- Calories: 260
- Protein: 18g
- Carbohydrates: 25g
- Fat: 10g
- Fiber: 8g

Directions:

- In a wok or skillet, heat sesame oil over medium-high heat.
- Add cubed tofu and stir-fry until golden.
- Add broccoli, red bell pepper, and julienned carrot.
- In a small bowl, mix teriyaki sauce and rice vinegar. Pour over the tofu and vegetables.
- Stir-fry until vegetables are crisp-tender.
- Garnish with sesame seeds and serve in a bowl.

Serving Methods:

1. Serve the teriyaki tofu stir-fry over brown rice for a fulfilling dinner.
2. Wrap the stir-fry in large lettuce leaves for a low-carb and refreshing option.

Spinach and Feta Stuffed Chicken Breast

Ingredients:

- 4 boneless, skinless chicken breasts
- 2 cups fresh spinach, wilted
- 1/2 cup feta cheese, crumbled
- 2 cloves garlic, minced
- 1 tablespoon olive oil

- 1 teaspoon dried oregano
- Salt and pepper to taste

Prep Time: 30 minutes

Cooking Time: 25 minutes

Serving Time: 55 minutes

Nutritional Info: (per serving)

- Calories: 320
- Protein: 30g
- Carbohydrates: 5g
- Fat: 18g
- Fiber: 2g

Directions:

- Preheat the oven to 375°F (190°C).
- In a skillet, sauté garlic in olive oil until fragrant.
- Add wilted spinach and cook until excess moisture evaporates.
- Butterfly each chicken breast and stuff with the spinach-feta mixture.
- Season with dried oregano, salt, and pepper.
- Bake for 25 minutes or until chicken is cooked through.
- Serve the stuffed chicken breasts on a plate.

Serving Methods:

1. Drizzle with balsamic reduction for an extra burst of flavor.
2. Pair with roasted Brussels sprouts or a side salad for a balanced and nutritious dinner.

Mediterranean Chickpea Salad

Ingredients: 2 cans (15 oz each) chickpeas, drained and rinsed

- 1 cucumber, diced
- 1 cup cherry tomatoes, halved
- 1/2 cup Kalamata olives, sliced
- 1/4 cup red onion, finely chopped
- 1/2 cup feta cheese, crumbled
- 3 tablespoons extra-virgin olive oil
- 2 tablespoons red wine vinegar
- 1 teaspoon dried oregano
- Salt and pepper to taste

Prep Time: 15 minutes

Serving Time: 15 minutes

Nutritional Info: (per serving)

- Calories: 280
- Protein: 10g
- Carbohydrates: 30g
- Fat: 15g
- Fiber: 8g

Directions: In a large bowl, combine chickpeas, cucumber, cherry tomatoes, olives, red onion, and feta cheese.

- In a small bowl, whisk together olive oil, red wine vinegar, dried oregano, salt, and pepper.
- Pour the dressing over the salad and toss to coat.
- Serve the Mediterranean chickpea salad on a plate.

Serving Methods:

1. Enjoy the salad as a light and refreshing dinner on its own.
2. Serve alongside grilled chicken or fish for added protein.

Cajun Shrimp and Quinoa Skillet

Ingredients: 1 lb shrimp, peeled and deveined

- 1 cup quinoa, cooked
- 1 bell pepper, diced
- 1/2 cup corn kernels
- 1/4 cup green onions, sliced
- 2 tablespoons Cajun seasoning
- 2 tablespoons olive oil
- Lemon wedges for serving

Prep Time: 20 minutes

Cooking Time: 15 minutes

Serving Time: 35 minutes

Nutritional Info: (per serving)

- Calories: 320
- Protein: 25g
- Carbohydrates: 30g
- Fat: 12g
- Fiber: 4g

Directions: In a skillet, heat olive oil over medium-high heat.

- Season shrimp with Cajun seasoning and cook until pink.
- Add diced bell pepper, corn, and cooked quinoa.
- Stir until well combined and heated through.
- Garnish with sliced green onions and serve on a plate.
- Squeeze lemon wedges over the dish before enjoying.

Serving Methods:

1. Pair the Cajun shrimp and quinoa skillet with a side of steamed broccoli.

2. Spoon the mixture into tortillas for a flavorful shrimp and quinoa wrap.

Caprese Stuffed Chicken Breast

Ingredients:

- 4 boneless, skinless chicken breasts
- 1 cup cherry tomatoes, sliced
- 1 cup fresh mozzarella, sliced
- 1/4 cup fresh basil leaves
- 2 tablespoons balsamic glaze
- 1 tablespoon olive oil
- Salt and pepper to taste

Prep Time: 20 minutes

Cooking Time: 25 minutes

Serving Time: 45 minutes

Nutritional Info: (per serving)

- Calories: 300
- Protein: 35g
- Carbohydrates: 5g
- Fat: 15g
- Fiber: 1g

Directions:

- Preheat the oven to 375°F (190°C).
- Butterfly each chicken breast and season with salt and pepper.
- Layer sliced cherry tomatoes, fresh mozzarella, and basil inside each chicken breast.
- Secure with toothpicks and place in a baking dish.
- Drizzle with olive oil and bake for 25 minutes or until chicken is cooked through.

- Drizzle with balsamic glaze before serving.

Serving Methods:

1. Serve the caprese stuffed chicken breast on a plate with a side of mixed greens.
2. Slice and arrange on a platter for an elegant and flavorful dinner.

Vegetarian Lentil and Mushroom Shepherd's Pie

Ingredients

- 3 cloves garlic, minced
- 1 teaspoon thyme
- 1 teaspoon rosemary
- 1/2 cup tomato paste
- 1 cup vegetable broth
- 4 cups mashed sweet potatoes
- Salt and pepper to taste
- 2 tablespoons olive oil

Prep Time: 30 minutes

Cooking Time: 40 minutes

Serving Time: 70 minutes

Nutritional Info: (per serving)

- Calories: 320
- Protein: 15g
- Carbohydrates: 55g
- Fat: 8g
- Fiber: 12g

Directions:

- Preheat the oven to 375°F (190°C).

- In a large skillet, heat olive oil over medium heat.
- Sauté onions, carrots, celery, and mushrooms until softened.
- Add minced garlic, thyme, and rosemary, stirring for an additional 2 minutes.
- Stir in cooked green lentils, tomato paste, and vegetable broth. Simmer for 10 minutes.
- Season with salt and pepper to taste.
- Transfer the lentil and mushroom mixture into a baking dish.
- Spread the mashed sweet potatoes evenly over the top.
- Bake for 30 minutes or until the top is golden brown.
- Allow it to cool for a few minutes before serving.

Serving Methods:

1. Serve generous portions of the vegetarian lentil and mushroom shepherd's pie on individual plates.
2. Pair it with a side salad for a well-balanced and hearty dinner.

Pesto Zoodles with Cherry Tomatoes and Grilled Chicken

Ingredients:

- 4 zucchinis, spiralized into zoodles
- 1 lb chicken breasts, grilled and sliced
- 1 cup cherry tomatoes, halved
- 1/2 cup basil pesto
- 1/4 cup pine nuts, toasted
- 2 tablespoons Parmesan cheese, grated
- Salt and pepper to taste

Prep Time: 20 minutes

Cooking Time: 15 minutes (for grilling chicken)

Serving Time: 35 minutes

Nutritional Info: (per serving)

- Calories: 280
- Protein: 30g
- Carbohydrates: 10g
- Fat: 15g
- Fiber: 3g

Directions:

- Spiralize the zucchinis into zoodles and set aside.
- Grill chicken breasts until fully cooked, then slice.
- In a large bowl, toss zoodles with cherry tomatoes, grilled chicken slices, and basil pesto.
- Top with toasted pine nuts and grated Parmesan cheese.
- Season with salt and pepper to taste.
- Serve the pesto zoodles with cherry tomatoes and grilled chicken on a plate.

Serving Methods:

1. Garnish with extra fresh basil for a burst of flavor.
2. Serve on a bed of arugula or mixed greens for added freshness.

SNACKS RECIPES

Greek Yogurt Parfait

Ingredients:

- 1 cup Greek yogurt
- 1/2 cup mixed berries (blueberries, strawberries)
- 1/4 cup granola
- 1 tablespoon honey
- 1 tablespoon chia seeds

Prep Time: 5 minutes

Serving Time: 5 minutes

Nutritional Info: (per serving)

- Calories: 250
- Protein: 15g
- Carbohydrates: 30g
- Fat: 8g
- Fiber: 5g

Directions:

- In a glass or bowl, layer Greek yogurt, mixed berries, and granola.
- Drizzle honey over the top and sprinkle with chia seeds.
- Serve the Greek yogurt parfait with a long spoon.

Serving Methods:

- Enjoy as a quick and nutritious mid-morning snack.

- Serve in small portable jars for an on-the-go snack.

Cucumber and Hummus Bites

Ingredients:

- 1 cucumber, sliced

- 1/2 cup hummus

- Cherry tomatoes, halved

- Fresh parsley for garnish

Prep Time: 10 minutes

Serving Time: 10 minutes

Nutritional Info: (per serving)

- Calories: 120

- Protein: 5g

- Carbohydrates: 15g

- Fat: 6g

- Fiber: 5g

Directions:

- Slice the cucumber into rounds.

- Top each cucumber slice with a dollop of hummus.

- Garnish with a cherry tomato half and fresh parsley.

- Serve the cucumber and hummus bites on a platter.

Serving Methods:

1. Arrange on a plate for a light afternoon snack.

2. Skewer the cucumber rounds and serve as a party appetizer.

Almond and Coconut Energy Balls

Ingredients

- 1 cup almonds, raw
- 1 cup dates, pitted
- 1/2 cup shredded coconut
- 1 tablespoon chia seeds
- 1 tablespoon almond butter
- 1 teaspoon vanilla extract

Prep Time: 15 minutes

Serving Time: 15 minutes

Nutritional Info: (per serving - 2 balls)

- Calories: 180
- Protein: 5g
- Carbohydrates: 20g
- Fat: 10g
- Fiber: 4g

Directions:

- In a food processor, combine almonds, dates, shredded coconut, chia seeds, almond butter, and vanilla extract.
- Pulse until the mixture forms a dough-like consistency.
- Roll the mixture into small balls.

- Refrigerate for 1 hour before serving.

Serving Methods:

1. Enjoy two almond and coconut energy balls as a snack between meals.

2. Pack in a small container for a convenient on-the-go energy boost.

Avocado and Tomato Salsa with Whole Grain Crackers

Ingredients:

- 1 avocado, diced

- 1 cup cherry tomatoes, diced

- 1/4 cup red onion, finely chopped

- 1/4 cup cilantro, chopped

- 1 lime, juiced

- Salt and pepper to taste

- Whole grain crackers

Prep Time: 10 minutes

Serving Time: 10 minutes

Nutritional Info: (per serving)

- Calories: 150

- Protein: 3g

- Carbohydrates: 20g

- Fat: 8g

- Fiber: 5g

Directions:

- In a bowl, combine diced avocado, cherry tomatoes, red onion, cilantro, lime juice, salt, and pepper.
- Mix gently to avoid mashing the avocado.
- Serve the avocado and tomato salsa with whole grain crackers.

Serving Methods:

1. Enjoy as a satisfying mid-afternoon snack.
2. Place the salsa in a small container and bring along with the crackers for a portable snack.

Berry and Nut Yogurt Bark

Ingredients:

- 2 cups Greek yogurt
- 1/2 cup mixed berries (strawberries, blueberries)
- 1/4 cup almonds, chopped
- 1 tablespoon honey
- 1 teaspoon vanilla extract

Prep Time: 10 minutes

Freezing Time: 4 hours

Serving Time: 5 minutes

Nutritional Info: (per serving)

- Calories: 180
- Protein: 15g

- Carbohydrates: 20g
- Fat: 6g
- Fiber: 2g

Directions:

- In a bowl, mix Greek yogurt, mixed berries, chopped almonds, honey, and vanilla extract.
- Line a baking sheet with parchment paper.
- Spread the yogurt mixture evenly on the parchment paper.
- Freeze for at least 4 hours or until firm.
- Break into pieces and serve the berry and nut yogurt bark.

Serving Methods:

1. Enjoy a couple of bark pieces as a cool and satisfying snack.
2. Top with additional fresh berries for an extra burst of flavor.

Quinoa and Vegetable Stuffed Bell Peppers

Ingredients:

- 2 bell peppers, halved and seeds removed
- 1 cup cooked quinoa
- 1/2 cup black beans, drained and rinsed
- 1/2 cup corn kernels
- 1/4 cup diced tomatoes
- 1/4 cup red onion, finely chopped
- 1 tablespoon lime juice
- 1 teaspoon cumin

- 1/2 teaspoon chili powder

- Fresh cilantro for garnish

Prep Time: 15 minutes

Serving Time: 15 minutes

Nutritional Info: (per serving)

- Calories: 180

- Protein: 6g

- Carbohydrates: 35g

- Fat: 2g

- Fiber: 6g

Directions:

- In a bowl, mix cooked quinoa, black beans, corn, diced tomatoes, red onion, lime juice, cumin, and chili powder.

- Spoon the mixture into halved bell peppers.

- Garnish with fresh cilantro and serve.

Serving Methods:

1. Enjoy the quinoa and vegetable stuffed bell peppers as a light and satisfying snack.

2. Serve with a side of salsa for added flavor.

Chocolate Avocado Mousse

Ingredients: 2 ripe avocados

- 1/4 cup unsweetened cocoa powder

- 1/4 cup maple syrup or honey
- 1 teaspoon vanilla extract
- Pinch of salt
- Fresh berries for garnish

Prep Time: 10 minutes

Chilling Time: 30 minutes

Serving Time: 5 minutes

Nutritional Info: (per serving)

- Calories: 200
- Protein: 3g
- Carbohydrates: 20g
- Fat: 15g
- Fiber: 8g

Directions:

- In a blender, combine ripe avocados, cocoa powder, maple syrup or honey, vanilla extract, and a pinch of salt.
- Blend until smooth and creamy.
- Chill in the refrigerator for at least 30 minutes.
- Garnish with fresh berries before serving.

Serving Methods:

1. Enjoy the chocolate avocado mousse as a guilt-free dessert-like snack.
2. Serve in small bowls or glasses for an elegant presentation.

Chia Seed Pudding with Almond Butter

Ingredients: 1/4 cup chia seeds, 1 cup almond milk

- 1 tablespoon almond butter
- 1 tablespoon maple syrup
- 1/2 teaspoon vanilla extract
- Sliced almonds for topping

Prep Time: 5 minutes

Chilling Time: 4 hours

Serving Time: 5 minutes

Nutritional Info: (per serving)

- Calories: 180
- Protein: 5g
- Carbohydrates: 15g
- Fat: 12g
- Fiber: 7g

Directions: In a bowl, mix chia seeds, almond milk, almond butter, maple syrup, and vanilla extract.

- Stir well and refrigerate for at least 4 hours or overnight.
- Top with sliced almonds before serving.

Serving Methods:

1. Enjoy the chia seed pudding with almond butter as a filling and nutritious snack.

2. Layer with fresh berries or banana slices for added sweetness.

Crispy Roasted Chickpeas

Ingredients:

- 1 can (15 oz) chickpeas, drained and rinsed
- 1 tablespoon olive oil
- 1 teaspoon smoked paprika
- 1/2 teaspoon cumin
- 1/2 teaspoon garlic powder
- Salt and pepper to taste

Prep Time: 10 minutes

Roasting Time: 30 minutes

Serving Time: 5 minutes

Nutritional Info: (per serving)

- Calories: 150
- Protein: 6g
- Carbohydrates: 20g
- Fat: 5g
- Fiber: 6g

Directions:

- Preheat the oven to 400°F (200°C).
- Pat the chickpeas dry with a paper towel.
- Toss chickpeas in olive oil, smoked paprika, cumin, garlic powder, salt, and pepper.

- Spread them on a baking sheet and roast for 30 minutes, shaking the pan halfway through.
- Allow to cool before serving.

Serving Methods:

1. Enjoy crispy roasted chickpeas as a crunchy and protein-packed snack.
2. Sprinkle with nutritional yeast for a cheesy flavor twist.

Mango and Cucumber Salsa with Baked Pita Chips

Ingredients:

- 1 ripe mango, diced
- 1 cucumber, peeled and diced
- 1/4 cup red onion, finely chopped
- 1 jalapeño, seeds removed and finely chopped
- 1/4 cup fresh cilantro, chopped
- Juice of 1 lime
- Baked whole wheat pita chips

Prep Time: 15 minutes

Serving Time: 10 minutes

Nutritional Info: (per serving)

- Calories: 120
- Protein: 2g
- Carbohydrates: 30g
- Fat: 1g

- Fiber: 4g

Directions:

- In a bowl, combine diced mango, cucumber, red onion, jalapeño, cilantro, and lime juice.
- Mix well and let it sit for flavors to meld.
- Serve with baked whole wheat pita chips.

Serving Methods:

1. Enjoy the mango and cucumber salsa as a refreshing snack.
2. Scoop the salsa into avocado halves for a creative and nutritious twist.

Egg Salad Stuffed Cucumber Boats

Ingredients:

- 2 cucumbers, halved lengthwise
- 4 hard-boiled eggs, chopped
- 2 tablespoons Greek yogurt
- 1 tablespoon Dijon mustard
- 1 tablespoon fresh dill, chopped
- Salt and pepper to taste
- Paprika for garnish

Prep Time: 15 minutes

Serving Time: 10 minutes

Nutritional Info: (per serving)

- Calories: 160
- Protein: 12g
- Carbohydrates: 5g
- Fat: 10g
- Fiber: 2g

Directions:

- Scoop out the seeds from the cucumber halves, creating a "boat" shape.
- In a bowl, mix chopped hard-boiled eggs, Greek yogurt, Dijon mustard, fresh dill, salt, and pepper.
- Spoon the egg salad into the cucumber boats.
- Sprinkle with paprika for a finishing touch.
- Serve the egg salad stuffed cucumber boats.

Serving Methods:

1. Enjoy as a light and protein-packed afternoon snack.
2. Serve on a platter for a delightful appetizer at gatherings.

Turmeric Roasted Nuts

Ingredients:

- 1 cup mixed nuts (almonds, walnuts, cashews)
- 1 tablespoon olive oil
- 1 teaspoon ground turmeric
- 1/2 teaspoon cayenne pepper
- 1 teaspoon honey

- Sea salt to taste

Prep Time: 10 minutes

Roasting Time: 15 minutes

Serving Time: 5 minutes

Nutritional Info: (per serving)

- Calories: 180
- Protein: 5g
- Carbohydrates: 6g
- Fat: 15g
- Fiber: 3g

Directions:

- Preheat the oven to 350°F (175°C).
- In a bowl, toss mixed nuts with olive oil, ground turmeric, cayenne pepper, honey, and a sprinkle of sea salt.
- Spread the nuts on a baking sheet and roast for 15 minutes, stirring halfway through.
- Allow to cool before serving.

Serving Methods:

1. Enjoy turmeric roasted nuts as a crunchy and anti-inflammatory snack.
2. Pack in small containers for a satisfying on-the-go snack.

Apple and Almond Butter Sandwiches

Ingredients:

- 1 apple, cored and sliced into rounds
- 2 tablespoons almond butter
- Granola for topping

Prep Time: 5 minutes

Serving Time: 5 minutes

Nutritional Info: (per serving)

- Calories: 200
- Protein: 5g
- Carbohydrates: 20g
- Fat: 12g
- Fiber: 5g

Directions:

- Spread almond butter on one side of each apple slice.
- Sprinkle granola on top of half of the apple slices.
- Sandwich the slices together with granola in the middle.
- Serve the apple and almond butter sandwiches.

Serving Methods

1. Enjoy as a sweet and satisfying mid-morning or afternoon snack.
2. Arrange on a plate for a visually appealing snack option.

Edamame and Sea Salt Pods

Ingredients: 2 cups edamame pods

- Sea salt to taste

Prep Time: 5 minutes

Cooking Time: 5 minutes

Serving Time: 5 minutes

Nutritional Info: (per serving)

- Calories: 150
- Protein: 12g
- Carbohydrates: 10g
- Fat: 8g
- Fiber: 6g

Directions: Boil or steam edamame pods according to package instructions.

- Sprinkle with sea salt while they are still warm.
- Serve the edamame pods in a bowl.

Serving Methods:

1. Enjoy as a protein-packed and satisfying snack.
2. Serve in a small bowl with a side of sea salt for dipping.

Coconut Chia Pudding with Mango

Ingredients: 1/4 cup chia seeds

- 1 cup coconut milk

- 1 tablespoon maple syrup

- 1/2 teaspoon vanilla extract

- 1/2 cup diced mango

Prep Time: 5 minutes

Chilling Time: 4 hours

Serving Time: 5 minutes

- *Nutritional Info:* (per serving)

- Calories: 180

- Protein: 4g

- Carbohydrates: 20g

- Fat: 10g

- Fiber: 8g

Directions: In a jar, mix chia seeds, coconut milk, maple syrup, and vanilla extract.

- Stir well and refrigerate for at least 4 hours or overnight.
- Top with diced mango before serving.

Serving Methods:

1. Enjoy coconut chia pudding as a creamy and tropical snack.
2. Layer with sliced kiwi or pineapple for added freshness.

Spinach and Feta Stuffed Mushrooms

Ingredients: 8 large mushrooms, stems removed

- 1 cup fresh spinach, chopped

- 1/2 cup feta cheese, crumbled
- 2 tablespoons olive oil, 1 clove garlic, minced
- Salt and pepper to taste
- Fresh parsley for garnish

Prep Time: 15 minutes

Cooking Time: 15 minutes

Serving Time: 5 minutes

Nutritional Info: (per serving)

- Calories: 120
- Protein: 5g
- Carbohydrates: 5g
- Fat: 10g
- Fiber: 2g

Directions: Preheat the oven to 375°F (190°C).

- In a skillet, sauté chopped spinach and minced garlic in olive oil until wilted.
- Stuff each mushroom with the spinach mixture and crumbled feta.
- Place on a baking sheet and bake for 15 minutes.
- Garnish with fresh parsley before serving.

Serving Methods:

1. Enjoy these spinach and feta stuffed mushrooms as a savory and satisfying snack.

2. Serve on a decorative platter for a sophisticated presentation at gatherings.

Protein-Packed Cottage Cheese and Pineapple Bowls

Ingredients:

- 1 cup low-fat cottage cheese
- 1 cup fresh pineapple chunks
- 2 tablespoons unsweetened coconut flakes
- 1 tablespoon honey
- Chopped mint leaves for garnish

Prep Time: 10 minutes

Serving Time: 5 minutes

Nutritional Info: (per serving)

- Calories: 180
- Protein: 15g
- Carbohydrates: 25g
- Fat: 5g
- Fiber: 3g

Directions:

- In a bowl, combine cottage cheese and fresh pineapple chunks.
- Sprinkle with coconut flakes and drizzle with honey.
- Garnish with chopped mint leaves and serve.

Serving Methods:

1. Enjoy as a protein-rich and tropical-flavored snack.
2. Serve in individual bowls for a quick and refreshing dessert.

Sweet Potato Toast with Almond Butter and Berries

Ingredients:

- 1 large sweet potato, sliced into 1/4-inch thick rounds
- 2 tablespoons almond butter
- Fresh berries (strawberries, blueberries)
- Chia seeds for topping

Prep Time: 10 minutes

Cooking Time: 15 minutes

Serving Time: 5 minutes

Nutritional Info: (per serving)

- Calories: 200
- Protein: 5g
- Carbohydrates: 30g
- Fat: 8g
- Fiber: 6g

Directions:

- Toast sweet potato rounds in a toaster or toaster oven until cooked through.
- Spread almond butter on each round.

- Top with fresh berries and sprinkle with chia seeds.

- Serve the sweet potato toast with almond butter and berries.

Serving Methods:

1. Enjoy as a nutrient-dense and satisfying snack.

2. Arrange on a plate for a visually appealing snack option.

Minty Watermelon Salad

Ingredients:

- 2 cups watermelon, diced

- 1/4 cup feta cheese, crumbled

- 1 tablespoon fresh mint, chopped

- 1 tablespoon balsamic glaze

- Black pepper to taste

Prep Time: 10 minutes

Serving Time: 5 minutes

Nutritional Info: (per serving)

- Calories: 90

- Protein: 2g

- Carbohydrates: 20g

- Fat: 2g

- Fiber: 1g

Directions: In a bowl, combine diced watermelon, crumbled feta, and chopped mint.

- Drizzle with balsamic glaze and sprinkle with black pepper.

- Gently toss and serve the minty watermelon salad.

Serving Methods:

1. Enjoy as a refreshing and hydrating snack.

2. Serve in individual bowls for a light and elegant dessert.

Sesame Ginger Edamame

Ingredients:

- 2 cups edamame, steamed or boiled

- 1 tablespoon sesame oil

- 1 tablespoon low-sodium soy sauce

- 1 teaspoon grated ginger

- Sesame seeds for garnish

Prep Time: 10 minutes

Cooking Time: 5 minutes

Serving Time: 5 minutes

Nutritional Info: (per serving)

- Calories: 150

- Protein: 14g

- Carbohydrates: 9g

- Fat: 8g

- Fiber: 4g

Directions: In a bowl, toss steamed or boiled edamame with sesame oil, soy sauce, and grated ginger.

- Garnish with sesame seeds before serving.

Serving Methods:

1. Enjoy sesame ginger edamame as a protein-packed and flavorful snack.
2. Serve in small bowls with toothpicks for a convenient and tasty appetizer.

SALAD RECIPES

Kale and Quinoa Power Salad

Ingredients:

- 2 cups kale, finely chopped
- 1 cup cooked quinoa
- 1/2 cup cherry tomatoes, halved
- 1/4 cup red onion, thinly sliced
- 1/4 cup feta cheese, crumbled
- 2 tablespoons olive oil
- 1 tablespoon balsamic vinegar
- Salt and pepper to taste
- Pumpkin seeds for garnish

Prep Time: 15 minutes

Serving Time: 5 minutes

Nutritional Info: (per serving)

- Calories: 280
- Protein: 10g
- Carbohydrates: 25g
- Fat: 15g
- Fiber: 5g

Directions:

- In a large bowl, combine chopped kale, cooked quinoa, cherry tomatoes, red onion, and feta cheese.

- Drizzle with olive oil and balsamic vinegar. Toss to coat.

- Season with salt and pepper to taste.

- Garnish with pumpkin seeds before serving.

Serving Methods:

1. Serve as a light lunch or dinner option.

2. Pack in a mason jar for a convenient and portable salad.

Mango Avocado Cilantro Lime Salad

Ingredients:

- 2 ripe avocados, diced

- 1 mango, diced

- 1/4 cup red onion, finely chopped

- 1/4 cup fresh cilantro, chopped

- Juice of 2 limes

- Salt and pepper to taste

- Mixed greens for the base

- Almonds for crunch

Prep Time: 10 minutes

Serving Time: 5 minutes

Nutritional Info: (per serving)

- Calories: 240

- Protein: 5g

- Carbohydrates: 20g

- Fat: 18g

- Fiber: 8g

Directions:

- In a bowl, combine diced avocados, mango, red onion, and cilantro.
- Squeeze lime juice over the mixture and toss gently.
- Season with salt and pepper to taste.
- Serve over a bed of mixed greens and top with almonds.

Serving Methods:

1. Enjoy as a refreshing and flavorful side salad.
2. Serve in avocado halves for a visually appealing and filling meal.

Caprese Salad with Balsamic Glaze

Ingredients:

- 2 cups cherry tomatoes, halved
- 1 cup fresh mozzarella, diced
- 1/4 cup fresh basil leaves
- 2 tablespoons balsamic glaze
- 1 tablespoon olive oil
- Salt and pepper to taste

Prep Time: 10 minutes

Serving Time: 5 minutes

Nutritional Info: (per serving)

- Calories: 220

- Protein: 10g

- Carbohydrates: 5g

- Fat: 18g

- Fiber: 1g

Directions:

- Arrange halved cherry tomatoes and diced mozzarella on a serving platter.

- Tuck fresh basil leaves among the tomatoes and mozzarella.

- Drizzle with balsamic glaze and olive oil.

- Season with salt and pepper to taste.

Serving Methods:

1. Serve as a classic and elegant appetizer.

2. Arrange on skewers for a bite-sized party option.

Asian-Inspired Salmon Salad

Ingredients:

- 1 lb grilled salmon, flaked

- 4 cups mixed salad greens

- 1 cup shredded cabbage

- 1/2 cup edamame, steamed

- 1/4 cup carrots, julienned

- 1/4 cup sliced cucumbers

- Sesame ginger dressing

- Sesame seeds for garnish

Prep Time: 20 minutes

Cooking Time: 10 minutes (for grilling salmon)

Serving Time: 5 minutes

Nutritional Info: (per serving)

- Calories: 320
- Protein: 25g
- Carbohydrates: 15g
- Fat: 18g
- Fiber: 6g

Directions:

- Grill salmon until fully cooked and flake into large pieces.
- In a large bowl, combine mixed salad greens, shredded cabbage, edamame, carrots, and sliced cucumbers.
- Add flaked salmon on top.
- Drizzle with sesame ginger dressing and toss gently.
- Garnish with sesame seeds before serving.

Serving Methods:

1. Serve as a substantial and protein-packed dinner salad.
2. Pack components separately for a refreshing and nutritious work lunch.

Mediterranean Chickpea Salad

Ingredients:

- 1 can (15 oz) chickpeas, drained and rinsed
- 1 cup cucumber, diced
- 1 cup cherry tomatoes, halved
- 1/2 cup red bell pepper, diced
- 1/4 cup red onion, finely chopped
- 1/4 cup feta cheese, crumbled
- 2 tablespoons olive oil
- Juice of 1 lemon
- 1 teaspoon dried oregano
- Salt and pepper to taste

Prep Time: 15 minutes

Serving Time: 5 minutes

Nutritional Info: (per serving)

- Calories: 280
- Protein: 10g
- Carbohydrates: 30g
- Fat: 15g
- Fiber: 8g

Directions: In a large bowl, combine chickpeas, cucumber, cherry tomatoes, red bell pepper, red onion, and feta cheese.

- Drizzle with olive oil and lemon juice. Sprinkle with dried oregano.
- Season with salt and pepper to taste. Toss gently.
- Serve the Mediterranean chickpea salad.

Serving Methods:

1. Enjoy as a hearty and flavorful lunch option.
2. Serve in pita pockets for a portable and satisfying meal.

Quinoa and Black Bean Fiesta Salad

Ingredients:

- 1 cup cooked quinoa
- 1 can (15 oz) black beans, drained and rinsed
- 1 cup corn kernels (fresh or thawed if frozen)
- 1 cup cherry tomatoes, quartered
- 1/4 cup red onion, finely chopped
- 1/4 cup cilantro, chopped
- Juice of 2 limes
- 2 tablespoons olive oil
- Cumin, chili powder, salt, and pepper to taste
- Avocado slices for garnish

Prep Time: 15 minutes

Serving Time: 5 minutes

Nutritional Info: (per serving)

- Calories: 280

- Protein: 10g

- Carbohydrates: 40g

- Fat: 10g

- Fiber: 8g

Directions:

- In a large bowl, combine cooked quinoa, black beans, corn, cherry tomatoes, red onion, and cilantro.

- In a small bowl, whisk together lime juice, olive oil, cumin, chili powder, salt, and pepper.

- Pour the dressing over the salad and toss gently.

- Garnish with avocado slices before serving.

Serving Methods:

1. Enjoy as a satisfying and protein-packed lunch.

2. Spoon into tortillas for a flavorful quinoa and black bean wrap.

Pear and Walnut Arugula Salad

Ingredients:

- 4 cups arugula

- 2 pears, sliced

- 1/2 cup walnuts, toasted

- 1/4 cup blue cheese, crumbled

- 2 tablespoons balsamic vinaigrette

- 1 tablespoon olive oil

- Salt and pepper to taste

Prep Time: 10 minutes

Serving Time: 5 minutes

Nutritional Info: (per serving)

- Calories: 220
- Protein: 5g
- Carbohydrates: 20g
- Fat: 15g
- Fiber: 4g

Directions:

- In a large salad bowl, combine arugula, sliced pears, toasted walnuts, and crumbled blue cheese.
- Drizzle with balsamic vinaigrette and olive oil.
- Season with salt and pepper to taste. Toss gently.
- Serve the pear and walnut arugula salad.

Serving Methods:

1. Enjoy as a light and sophisticated side salad.
2. Top with grilled chicken for a complete and filling meal.

Tuna and Chickpea Salad Bowl

Ingredients:

- 1 can (5 oz) tuna, drained
- 1 cup chickpeas, drained and rinsed
- 1 cucumber, diced
- 1/2 cup cherry tomatoes, halved

- 1/4 cup red onion, finely chopped
- 2 tablespoons Greek yogurt
- 1 tablespoon Dijon mustard
- Juice of 1 lemon
- Salt and pepper to taste
- Fresh parsley for garnish

Prep Time: 15 minutes

Serving Time: 5 minutes

Nutritional Info: (per serving)

- Calories: 280
- Protein: 25g
- Carbohydrates: 25g
- Fat: 10g
- Fiber: 8g

Directions: In a large bowl, mix tuna, chickpeas, cucumber, cherry tomatoes, and red onion.

- In a small bowl, whisk together Greek yogurt, Dijon mustard, and lemon juice.
- Pour the dressing over the salad and toss gently.
- Season with salt and pepper to taste.
- ***Garnish with fresh parsley before serving.***

Serving Methods:

1. Enjoy as a protein-rich and satisfying lunch.

2. Serve on a bed of mixed greens for an extra boost of nutrients.

Broccoli and Cranberry Quinoa Salad

Ingredients:

- 2 cups cooked quinoa
- 2 cups broccoli florets, blanched
- 1/2 cup dried cranberries
- 1/4 cup red onion, finely chopped
- 1/4 cup feta cheese, crumbled
- 2 tablespoons olive oil
- 1 tablespoon apple cider vinegar
- 1 teaspoon honey
- Salt and pepper to taste

Prep Time: 15 minutes

Serving Time: 5 minutes

Nutritional Info: (per serving)

- Calories: 250
- Protein: 8g
- Carbohydrates: 30g
- Fat: 12g
- Fiber: 5g

Directions:

- In a large bowl, combine cooked quinoa, blanched broccoli, dried cranberries, red onion, and feta cheese.

- In a small bowl, whisk together olive oil, apple cider vinegar, honey, salt, and pepper.
- Pour the dressing over the salad and toss gently.
- Serve the broccoli and cranberry quinoa salad.

Serving Methods:

1. Enjoy as a colorful and nutritious side dish.
2. Top with grilled shrimp for a protein-packed main course.

Greek Chicken Salad with Tzatziki Dressing

Ingredients:

- 1 lb grilled chicken, sliced
- 4 cups mixed salad greens
- 1 cup cherry tomatoes, halved
- 1 cucumber, sliced
- 1/4 cup red onion, thinly sliced
- 1/4 cup Kalamata olives, pitted
- 1/4 cup feta cheese, crumbled
- Tzatziki dressing
- Fresh oregano for garnish

Prep Time: 20 minutes

Cooking Time: 15 minutes (for grilling chicken)

Serving Time: 5 minutes

Nutritional Info: (per serving)

- Calories: 320

- Protein: 30g
- Carbohydrates: 15g
- Fat: 18g
- Fiber: 5g

Directions:

- Grill chicken until fully cooked and slice into strips.
- In a large bowl, combine mixed salad greens, cherry tomatoes, cucumber, red onion, olives, and feta cheese.
- Add grilled chicken on top.
- Drizzle with tzatziki dressing and toss gently.
- Garnish with fresh oregano before serving.

Serving Methods:

1. Enjoy as a satisfying and protein-packed dinner salad.
2. Serve in whole-grain pita pockets for a Greek-inspired wrap.

Spinach and Strawberry Salad with Poppy Seed Dressing

Ingredients:

- 4 cups baby spinach
- 1 cup strawberries, sliced
- 1/4 cup red onion, thinly sliced
- 1/4 cup goat cheese, crumbled
- 1/4 cup almonds, sliced and toasted
- Poppy seed dressing
- Balsamic glaze for drizzling

Prep Time: 10 minutes

Serving Time: 5 minutes

Nutritional Info: (per serving)

- Calories: 220
- Protein: 8g
- Carbohydrates: 15g
- Fat: 15g
- Fiber: 4g

Directions:

- In a large bowl, combine baby spinach, sliced strawberries, red onion, goat cheese, and toasted almonds.
- Drizzle with poppy seed dressing and toss gently.
- Drizzle with balsamic glaze before serving.

Serving Methods:

1. Enjoy as a light and refreshing lunch salad.
2. Serve in individual bowls for an elegant side dish.

Shrimp and Avocado Cobb Salad

Ingredients:

- 1 lb grilled shrimp, peeled and deveined
- 4 cups Romaine lettuce, chopped
- 1 cup cherry tomatoes, halved
- 1 avocado, diced
- 4 hard-boiled eggs, sliced

- 1/2 cup bacon bits
- Blue cheese crumbles
- Ranch dressing

Prep Time: 20 minutes

Cooking Time: 10 minutes (for grilling shrimp and boiling eggs)

Serving Time: 5 minutes

Nutritional Info: (per serving)

- Calories: 350
- Protein: 30g
- Carbohydrates: 15g
- Fat: 20g
- Fiber: 6g

Directions:

- Grill shrimp until fully cooked.
- In a large bowl, arrange chopped Romaine lettuce, cherry tomatoes, diced avocado, sliced hard-boiled eggs, and grilled shrimp.
- Sprinkle with bacon bits and blue cheese crumbles.
- Drizzle with ranch dressing before serving.

Serving Methods:

1. Enjoy as a hearty and protein-rich dinner salad.
2. Serve on a large platter for a festive gathering.

Roasted Beet and Goat Cheese Salad

Ingredients:

- 3 medium beets, roasted and sliced

- 4 cups arugula

- 1/4 cup walnuts, chopped and toasted

- 1/4 cup goat cheese, crumbled

- Balsamic vinaigrette

- Fresh thyme for garnish

Prep Time: 15 minutes

Cooking Time: 45 minutes (for roasting beets)

Serving Time: 5 minutes

Nutritional Info: (per serving)

- Calories: 250

- Protein: 8g

- Carbohydrates: 20g

- Fat: 15g

- Fiber: 6g

Directions:

- Roast beets until tender, peel, and slice.

- In a large bowl, combine arugula, roasted beets, toasted walnuts, and goat cheese.

- Drizzle with balsamic vinaigrette and toss gently.

- Garnish with fresh thyme before serving.

Serving Methods:

1. Enjoy as an elegant and flavorful side salad.
2. Serve on a bed of quinoa for a wholesome main course.

Cauliflower and Broccoli Detox Salad

Ingredients:

- 2 cups cauliflower florets, blanched
- 2 cups broccoli florets, blanched
- 1/2 cup red cabbage, thinly sliced
- 1/4 cup sunflower seeds, toasted
- 2 tablespoons tahini dressing
- Juice of 1 lemon
- Salt and pepper to taste

Prep Time: 15 minutes

Cooking Time: 5 minutes (for blanching)

Serving Time: 5 minutes

Nutritional Info: (per serving)

- Calories: 180
- Protein: 8g
- Carbohydrates: 15g
- Fat: 10g
- Fiber: 6g

Directions: Blanch cauliflower and broccoli florets until slightly tender.

- In a large bowl, combine blanched cauliflower and broccoli, sliced red cabbage, and toasted sunflower seeds.

- Drizzle with tahini dressing and lemon juice. Toss gently.

- Season with salt and pepper to taste.

Serving Methods:

1. Enjoy as a crunchy and detoxifying lunch option.
2. Serve in lettuce cups for a low-carb alternative.

Mango and Quinoa Summer Salad

Ingredients:

- 1 cup cooked quinoa

- 1 mango, diced

- 1 cucumber, diced

- 1/4 cup red bell pepper, diced

- 1/4 cup fresh cilantro, chopped

- Lime vinaigrette

- Tajin seasoning for a kick

Prep Time: 15 minutes

Serving Time: 5 minutes

Nutritional Info: (per serving)

- Calories: 220

- Protein: 6g

- Carbohydrates: 35g

- Fat: 5g

- Fiber: 5g

Directions:

- In a large bowl, combine cooked quinoa, diced mango, diced cucumber, diced red bell pepper, and chopped cilantro.
- Drizzle with lime vinaigrette and toss gently.
- Sprinkle with Tajin seasoning for a spicy kick.

Serving Methods:

1. Enjoy as a tropical and satisfying side salad.
2. Serve in a hollowed-out pineapple for a visually appealing presentation.

Grilled Chicken and Berry Salad

Ingredients:

- 1 lb grilled chicken breast, sliced
- 4 cups mixed salad greens
- 1 cup strawberries, sliced
- 1/2 cup blueberries
- 1/4 cup red onion, thinly sliced
- Feta cheese, crumbled
- Raspberry vinaigrette
- Chopped mint for garnish

Prep Time: 20 minutes

Cooking Time: 15 minutes (for grilling chicken)

Serving Time: 5 minutes

Nutritional Info: (per serving)

- Calories: 300
- Protein: 30g
- Carbohydrates: 20g
- Fat: 12g
- Fiber: 5g

Directions:

- Grill chicken until fully cooked and slice into strips.
- In a large bowl, combine mixed salad greens, sliced strawberries, blueberries, and red onion.
- Add grilled chicken on top.
- Sprinkle with crumbled feta cheese.
- Drizzle with raspberry vinaigrette and toss gently.
- Garnish with chopped mint before serving.

Serving Methods:

1. Enjoy as a protein-packed and refreshing dinner salad.
2. Serve on individual plates for an elegant presentation.

Asian Sesame Chicken Salad

Ingredients:

- 1 lb grilled chicken, sliced
- 4 cups Napa cabbage, shredded
- 1 cup snow peas, sliced
- 1/2 cup carrots, julienned

- 1/4 cup green onions, chopped
- 1/4 cup almonds, sliced and toasted
- Sesame ginger dressing
- Sesame seeds for garnish

Prep Time: 20 minutes

Cooking Time: 15 minutes (for grilling chicken)

Serving Time: 5 minutes

Nutritional Info: (per serving)

- Calories: 280
- Protein: 25g
- Carbohydrates: 15g
- Fat: 15g
- Fiber: 5g

Directions:

- Grill chicken until fully cooked and slice into strips.
- In a large bowl, combine shredded Napa cabbage, sliced snow peas, julienned carrots, green onions, and toasted almonds.
- Add grilled chicken on top.
- Drizzle with sesame ginger dressing and toss gently.
- Garnish with sesame seeds before serving.

Serving Methods:

1. Enjoy as a flavorful and satisfying lunch salad.

2. Serve in takeout containers for a convenient and healthy meal on the go.

Sun-Dried Tomato and Basil Quinoa Salad

Ingredients:

- 2 cups cooked quinoa
- 1/2 cup sun-dried tomatoes, chopped
- 1/4 cup fresh basil, chopped
- 1/4 cup black olives, sliced
- 1/4 cup feta cheese, crumbled
- Lemon vinaigrette
- Pine nuts for garnish

Prep Time: 15 minutes

Serving Time: 5 minutes

Nutritional Info: (per serving)

- Calories: 250
- Protein: 8g
- Carbohydrates: 30g
- Fat: 10g
- Fiber: 5g

Directions:

- In a large bowl, combine cooked quinoa, chopped sun-dried tomatoes, fresh basil, sliced black olives, and crumbled feta cheese.

- Drizzle with lemon vinaigrette and toss gently.
- Garnish with pine nuts before serving.

Serving Methods:

1. Enjoy as a Mediterranean-inspired side salad.
2. Serve in chilled bowls for a refreshing summer dish.

Brussels Sprouts and Pomegranate Salad

Ingredients:

- 4 cups Brussels sprouts, shaved
- 1/2 cup pomegranate seeds
- 1/4 cup pecans, chopped and toasted
- 1/4 cup Parmesan cheese, shaved
- Balsamic vinaigrette
- Dijon mustard for dressing
- Salt and pepper to taste

Prep Time: 15 minutes

Serving Time: 5 minutes

Nutritional Info: (per serving)

- Calories: 220
- Protein: 10g
- Carbohydrates: 20g
- Fat: 15g
- Fiber: 8g

Directions: Shave Brussels sprouts using a mandoline or sharp knife.

- In a large bowl, combine shaved Brussels sprouts, pomegranate seeds, toasted pecans, and shaved Parmesan cheese.

- In a small bowl, whisk together balsamic vinaigrette, Dijon mustard, salt, and pepper.

- Pour the dressing over the salad and toss gently.

Serving Methods:

1. Enjoy as a crunchy and festive holiday side dish.
2. Serve in a large salad bowl for family gatherings.

Mexican Street Corn Salad

Ingredients:

- 4 cups corn kernels, grilled or roasted
- 1/4 cup mayonnaise
- 1/4 cup sour cream
- 1/4 cup cotija cheese, crumbled
- 2 tablespoons fresh cilantro, chopped
- 1 teaspoon chili powder
- Lime wedges for serving

Prep Time: 15 minutes

Cooking Time: 10 minutes (for grilling or roasting corn)

Serving Time: 5 minutes

Nutritional Info: (per serving)

- Calories: 230
- Protein: 5g

- Carbohydrates: 30g
- Fat: 12g
- Fiber: 4g

Directions:

- Grill or roast corn until kernels are slightly charred.
- In a large bowl, combine grilled corn, mayonnaise, sour cream, crumbled cotija cheese, chopped cilantro, and chili powder.
- Toss gently until well coated.
- Serve the Mexican street corn salad with lime wedges.

Serving Methods:

1. Enjoy as a flavorful and savory side dish.
2. Serve in individual cups for a fun and interactive appetizer.

DESSERTS RECIPES

Chia Seed Pudding with Berries

Ingredients:

- 1/4 cup chia seeds
- 1 cup unsweetened almond milk
- 1 teaspoon vanilla extract
- Mixed berries (blueberries, strawberries, raspberries)
- 1 tablespoon honey or maple syrup (optional)

Prep Time: 5 minutes

Cooking Time: 0 minutes

Serving Time: 4 hours (chilling time)

Nutritional Info: (per serving)

- Calories: 150
- Protein: 5g
- Carbohydrates: 15g
- Fat: 8g
- Fiber: 7g

Directions:

- In a bowl, mix chia seeds, almond milk, and vanilla extract. Stir well.
- Cover and refrigerate for at least 4 hours or overnight.
- Before serving, layer chia pudding with mixed berries.

- Drizzle with honey or maple syrup if desired.

Serving Methods:

1. Serve in individual jars for a portion-controlled treat.
2. Top with a dollop of Greek yogurt for added creaminess.

Avocado Chocolate Mousse

Ingredients:

- 2 ripe avocados
- 1/4 cup unsweetened cocoa powder
- 1/4 cup maple syrup
- 1 teaspoon vanilla extract
- Pinch of salt
- Berries for garnish

Prep Time: 10 minutes

Cooking Time: 0 minutes

Serving Time: 2 hours (chilling time)

Nutritional Info: (per serving)

- Calories: 200
- Protein: 3g
- Carbohydrates: 20g
- Fat: 15g
- Fiber: 8g

Directions: In a food processor, blend avocados, cocoa powder, maple syrup, vanilla extract, and a pinch of salt until smooth.

- Refrigerate for at least 2 hours.
- Before serving, spoon the avocado chocolate mousse into bowls.
- Garnish with fresh berries.

Serving Methods:

1. Serve in elegant dessert glasses for a refined presentation.
2. Top with a dollop of whipped coconut cream for a decadent touch.

Baked Apples with Cinnamon and Walnuts

Ingredients:

- 4 medium apples, cored and halved
- 1 tablespoon lemon juice
- 2 tablespoons chopped walnuts
- 1 teaspoon cinnamon
- 1 tablespoon honey
- Greek yogurt for serving

Prep Time: 10 minutes

Cooking Time: 30 minutes

Serving Time: 5 minutes

Nutritional Info: (per serving)

- Calories: 180
- Protein: 3g
- Carbohydrates: 30g
- Fat: 8g
- Fiber: 6g

Directions:

- Preheat the oven to 350°F (180°C).
- Place apple halves in a baking dish and drizzle with lemon juice.
- In a small bowl, mix chopped walnuts, cinnamon, and honey.
- Spoon the mixture onto each apple half.
- Bake for 30 minutes or until apples are tender.
- Serve warm with a side of Greek yogurt.

Serving Methods:

1. Enjoy as a warm dessert straight from the oven.
2. Top with a sprinkle of granola for added crunch.

Coconut Almond Energy Bites

Ingredients:

- 1 cup shredded coconut
- 1/2 cup almond flour
- 1/4 cup almond butter
- 2 tablespoons coconut oil, melted
- 1 tablespoon honey

- 1 teaspoon vanilla extract

- Dark chocolate chips for coating

Prep Time: 15 minutes

Cooking Time: 0 minutes

Serving Time: 1 hour (chilling time)

Nutritional Info: (per serving)

- Calories: 120

- Protein: 2g

- Carbohydrates: 8g

- Fat: 9g

- Fiber: 3g

Directions:

- In a bowl, combine shredded coconut, almond flour, almond butter, melted coconut oil, honey, and vanilla extract.

- Mix until well combined.

- Form the mixture into small energy bites.

- Melt dark chocolate and dip each energy bite to coat.

- Place in the refrigerator for at least 1 hour before serving.

Serving Methods:

1. Serve on a decorative platter for a party dessert.

2. Pack in airtight containers for a portable and energizing snack.

Greek Yogurt Parfait with Mixed Berries

Ingredients:

- 1 cup Greek yogurt
- 1/2 cup mixed berries (blueberries, strawberries, raspberries)
- 1/4 cup granola
- 1 tablespoon honey
- Mint leaves for garnish

Prep Time: 5 minutes

Cooking Time: 0 minutes

Serving Time: 5 minutes

Nutritional Info: (per serving)

- Calories: 180
- Protein: 15g
- Carbohydrates: 25g
- Fat: 4g
- Fiber: 3g

Directions: In a glass or bowl, layer Greek yogurt, mixed berries, and granola.

- Drizzle with honey.
- Garnish with mint leaves before serving.

Serving Methods:

1. Serve in individual glasses for a visually appealing dessert.

2. Top with a sprinkle of chia seeds for added texture.

Almond Butter Banana Bites

Ingredients:

- 2 bananas, sliced
- 1/4 cup almond butter
- 2 tablespoons dark chocolate chips
- Crushed almonds for coating

Prep Time: 10 minutes

Cooking Time: 0 minutes

Serving Time: 30 minutes (freezing time)

Nutritional Info: (per serving)

- Calories: 140
- Protein: 3g
- Carbohydrates: 18g
- Fat: 7g
- Fiber: 3g

Directions: Spread almond butter on banana slices.

- Create banana sandwiches and dip each in dark chocolate.
- Roll in crushed almonds.
- Place on a tray and freeze for at least 30 minutes before serving.

Serving Methods:

1. Serve as a frozen, guilt-free dessert.

2. Arrange on a platter for a quick and healthy party treat.

Raspberry Chia Jam Thumbprint Cookies

Ingredients:

- 1 cup almond flour
- 2 tablespoons coconut oil, melted
- 2 tablespoons maple syrup
- Raspberry chia jam
- Fresh raspberries for garnish

Prep Time: 15 minutes

Cooking Time: 12 minutes

Serving Time: 5 minutes

Nutritional Info: (per serving)

- Calories: 120
- Protein: 2g
- Carbohydrates: 10g
- Fat: 8g
- Fiber: 3g

Directions:

- Preheat the oven to 350°F (180°C).
- In a bowl, mix almond flour, melted coconut oil, and maple syrup.
- Form small dough balls and press with your thumb to create a well.

- Spoon raspberry chia jam into the well.

- Bake for 12 minutes.

- Garnish with fresh raspberries before serving.

Serving Methods:

1. Serve as a wholesome afternoon snack.

2. Arrange on a plate for a tea-time dessert.

Mint Chocolate Avocado Popsicles

Ingredients:

- 2 ripe avocados

- 1/4 cup cocoa powder

- 1/4 cup fresh mint leaves

- 1/4 cup honey or maple syrup

- Dark chocolate drizzle

Prep Time: 10 minutes

Freezing Time: 4 hours

Serving Time: 5 minutes

Nutritional Info: (per serving)

- Calories: 160

- Protein: 2g

- Carbohydrates: 20g

- Fat: 9g

- Fiber: 5g

Directions:

- In a blender, combine avocados, cocoa powder, fresh mint, and honey.
- Blend until smooth.
- Pour into popsicle molds and freeze for at least 4 hours.
- Drizzle with melted dark chocolate before serving.

Serving Methods:

1. Serve as a refreshing dessert on a hot day.
2. Offer as a guilt-free treat during gatherings.

Peach and Almond Yogurt Parfait

Ingredients:

- 1 cup Greek yogurt
- 1 peach, sliced
- 2 tablespoons almond slices, toasted
- 1 tablespoon honey
- Cinnamon for sprinkling

Prep Time: 5 minutes

Cooking Time: 5 minutes (for toasting almonds)

Serving Time: 5 minutes

Nutritional Info: (per serving)

- Calories: 180
- Protein: 15g

- Carbohydrates: 20g

- Fat: 5g

- Fiber: 3g

Directions:

- In a glass or bowl, layer Greek yogurt and sliced peaches.

- Drizzle with honey.

- Sprinkle toasted almond slices and cinnamon before serving.

Serving Methods:

1. Serve in elegant dessert bowls for a sophisticated touch.

2. Top with a scoop of vanilla ice cream for a decadent treat.

Blueberry Lemon Cheesecake Bites

Ingredients:

- 1 cup cashews, soaked overnight

- 1/4 cup coconut oil, melted

- 1/4 cup maple syrup

- Zest and juice of 1 lemon

- 1/2 cup blueberries

- Graham cracker crumbs for coating

Prep Time: 15 minutes

Freezing Time: 3 hours

Serving Time: 5 minutes

Nutritional Info: (per serving)

- Calories: 160
- Protein: 3g
- Carbohydrates: 15g
- Fat: 10g
- Fiber: 2g

Directions:

- In a food processor, blend soaked cashews, melted coconut oil, maple syrup, lemon zest, and lemon juice until smooth.
- Spoon the mixture into mini muffin cups.
- Drop a few blueberries into each cup and swirl with a toothpick.
- Sprinkle graham cracker crumbs on top.
- Freeze for at least 3 hours before serving.

Serving Methods:

1. Serve as a mini cheesecake for individual indulgence.
2. Arrange on a dessert platter for a dinner party.

Cinnamon Baked Pears

Ingredients:

- 4 ripe pears, halved and cored
- 1 tablespoon coconut oil, melted
- 1 teaspoon cinnamon
- 2 tablespoons chopped walnuts
- 1 tablespoon honey

Prep Time: 10 minutes

Cooking Time: 25 minutes

Serving Time: 5 minutes

Nutritional Info: (per serving)

- Calories: 150

- Protein: 2g

- Carbohydrates: 20g

- Fat: 8g

- Fiber: 6g

Directions:

- Preheat the oven to 375°F (190°C).

- Place pear halves on a baking sheet.

- Drizzle with melted coconut oil and sprinkle with cinnamon.

- Roast for 25 minutes or until pears are tender.

- Top with chopped walnuts and a drizzle of honey before serving.

Serving Methods:

1. Serve warm as a comforting dessert.

2. Pair with a scoop of low-fat vanilla ice cream for an extra treat.

Strawberry Frozen Yogurt Popsicles

Ingredients:

- 2 cups fresh strawberries, hulled

- 1 cup Greek yogurt

- 2 tablespoons honey

- 1 teaspoon vanilla extract

Prep Time: 10 minutes

Freezing Time: 4 hours

Serving Time: 5 minutes

Nutritional Info: (per serving)

- Calories: 100

- Protein: 5g

- Carbohydrates: 15g

- Fat: 2g

- Fiber: 2g

Directions:

- In a blender, combine strawberries, Greek yogurt, honey, and vanilla extract.

- Blend until smooth.

- Pour the mixture into popsicle molds and freeze for at least 4 hours.

- Run molds under warm water to release the popsicles before serving.

Serving Methods:

1. Enjoy as a refreshing and guilt-free summer dessert.
2. Dip in dark chocolate for an indulgent twist.

Pumpkin Spice Chia Pudding

Ingredients:

- 1/4 cup chia seeds
- 1 cup unsweetened almond milk
- 1/4 cup canned pumpkin puree
- 1 tablespoon maple syrup
- 1/2 teaspoon pumpkin spice blend

Prep Time: 5 minutes

Chilling Time: 4 hours

Serving Time: 5 minutes

Nutritional Info: (per serving)

- Calories: 120
- Protein: 3g
- Carbohydrates: 15g
- Fat: 5g
- Fiber: 8g

Directions: In a bowl, mix chia seeds, almond milk, pumpkin puree, maple syrup, and pumpkin spice blend. Stir well.

- Cover and refrigerate for at least 4 hours or overnight.
- Before serving, top with a sprinkle of additional pumpkin spice.

Serving Methods:

1. Serve in festive dessert bowls during fall.

2. Garnish with a dollop of whipped coconut cream for added richness.

Chocolate Avocado Mousse Parfait

Ingredients:

- 2 ripe avocados
- 1/4 cup cocoa powder
- 1/4 cup maple syrup
- 1 teaspoon vanilla extract
- Granola for layering
- Fresh berries for topping

Prep Time: 10 minutes

Chilling Time: 2 hours

Serving Time: 5 minutes

Nutritional Info: (per serving)

- Calories: 180
- Protein: 3g
- Carbohydrates: 25g
- Fat: 10g
- Fiber: 7g

Directions:

- In a blender, combine avocados, cocoa powder, maple syrup, and vanilla extract.
- Blend until smooth.

- Layer the chocolate avocado mousse with granola in glasses.

- Refrigerate for at least 2 hours.

- Top with fresh berries before serving.

Serving Methods:

1. Serve as a decadent dessert parfait.

2. Garnish with a sprig of mint for an elegant touch.

Mango Coconut Chia Popsicles

Ingredients:

- 1 cup fresh mango, diced

- 1 cup coconut water

- 2 tablespoons chia seeds

- 1 tablespoon agave nectar or honey

Prep Time: 10 minutes

Freezing Time: 4 hours

Serving Time: 5 minutes

Nutritional Info: (per serving)

- Calories: 80

- Protein: 2g

- Carbohydrates: 15g

- Fat: 2g

- Fiber: 4g

Directions: In a blender, combine fresh mango and coconut water. Blend until smooth.

- Stir in chia seeds and agave nectar.
- Pour the mixture into popsicle molds and freeze for at least 4 hours.
- Run molds under warm water to release the popsicles before serving.

Serving Methods:

1. Enjoy as a tropical and hydrating frozen treat.
2. Dip in shredded coconut for an extra layer of flavor.

Cocoa Almond Energy Bites

Ingredients:

- 1 cup rolled oats
- 1/2 cup almond butter
- 1/4 cup cocoa powder
- 1/4 cup honey
- 1 teaspoon vanilla extract
- Shredded coconut for rolling

Prep Time: 15 minutes

Chilling Time: 1 hour

Serving Time: 5 minutes

Nutritional Info: (per serving)

- Calories: 140
- Protein: 5g
- Carbohydrates: 15g
- Fat: 8g
- Fiber: 3g

Directions:

- In a bowl, mix rolled oats, almond butter, cocoa powder, honey, and vanilla extract.
- Form the mixture into small energy bites.
- Roll in shredded coconut.
- Chill in the refrigerator for at least 1 hour before serving.

Serving Methods:

1. Serve as a quick energy-boosting dessert.
2. Package in small containers for an on-the-go snack.

Pineapple Coconut Sorbet

Ingredients:

- 2 cups frozen pineapple chunks
- 1/2 cup coconut milk
- 1 tablespoon lime juice
- Fresh mint for garnish

Prep Time: 5 minutes

Freezing Time: 4 hours

Serving Time: 5 minutes

Nutritional Info: (per serving)

- Calories: 90
- Protein: 1g
- Carbohydrates: 20g
- Fat: 2g
- Fiber: 2g

Directions:

- In a blender, combine frozen pineapple chunks, coconut milk, and lime juice.
- Blend until smooth.
- Transfer to a shallow dish and freeze for at least 4 hours.
- Scoop into bowls and garnish with fresh mint before serving.

Serving Methods:

1. Enjoy as a light and refreshing tropical dessert.
2. Serve in chilled bowls for a summer treat.

Vanilla Berry Parfait

Ingredients:

- 1 cup low-fat vanilla yogurt
- Mixed berries (strawberries, blueberries, raspberries)
- Granola for layering
- 1 tablespoon honey

Prep Time: 5 minutes

Serving Time: 5 minutes

Nutritional Info: (per serving)

- Calories: 160
- Protein: 8g
- Carbohydrates: 25g
- Fat: 3g
- Fiber: 4g

Directions:

- In a glass or bowl, layer low-fat vanilla yogurt, mixed berries, and granola.
- Drizzle with honey before serving.

Serving Methods:

1. Serve as a delightful and nutritious breakfast dessert.
2. Top with a sprinkle of crushed nuts for added crunch.

Coconut Lime Rice Pudding

Ingredients:

- 1 cup cooked brown rice
- 1 cup light coconut milk
- 2 tablespoons honey or agave nectar
- Zest and juice of 1 lime
- Toasted coconut flakes for garnish

Prep Time: 10 minutes

Cooking Time: 15 minutes

Serving Time: 5 minutes

Nutritional Info: (per serving)

- Calories: 180
- Protein: 3g
- Carbohydrates: 30g
- Fat: 5g
- Fiber: 2g

Directions:

- In a saucepan, combine cooked brown rice, coconut milk, honey or agave nectar, lime zest, and lime juice.
- Simmer over low heat for 15 minutes, stirring occasionally.
- Let it cool slightly before serving.
- Garnish with toasted coconut flakes.

Serving Methods:

1. Serve as a tropical twist on classic rice pudding.
2. Spoon into individual cups for a charming presentation.

Banana Nut Oat Cookies

- ***Ingredients:***
- 2 ripe bananas, mashed
- 1 cup rolled oats
- 1/4 cup chopped walnuts
- 1/4 cup raisins
- 1 teaspoon cinnamon

- 1 teaspoon vanilla extract

Prep Time: 10 minutes

Baking Time: 15 minutes

Serving Time: 5 minutes

Nutritional Info: (per serving)

- Calories: 120
- Protein: 3g
- Carbohydrates: 20g
- Fat: 4g
- Fiber: 3g

Directions:

- Preheat the oven to 350°F (180°C).
- In a bowl, mix mashed bananas, rolled oats, chopped walnuts, raisins, cinnamon, and vanilla extract.
- Drop spoonfuls of the mixture onto a baking sheet.
- Bake for 15 minutes or until golden brown.
- Allow to cool before serving.

Serving Methods:

1. Serve as a wholesome cookie alternative.
2. Enjoy with a cup of herbal tea for a cozy dessert.

MEAT AND POULTRY RECIPES

Grilled Lemon Herb Chicken Breast

Ingredients:

- 4 boneless, skinless chicken breasts
- 2 lemons (zested and juiced)
- 2 tablespoons olive oil
- 2 cloves garlic, minced
- 1 teaspoon dried oregano
- Salt and pepper to taste

Prep Time: 15 minutes

Cooking Time: 15 minutes

Serving Time: 5 minutes

Nutritional Info: (per serving)

- Calories: 200
- Protein: 25g
- Carbohydrates: 2g
- Fat: 10g
- Fiber: 1g

Directions:

- In a bowl, mix lemon zest, lemon juice, olive oil, minced garlic, dried oregano, salt, and pepper to create a marinade.

- Coat chicken breasts with the marinade and let them sit for at least 30 minutes.

- Grill chicken for about 7-8 minutes per side or until cooked through.

- Serve with a side of steamed vegetables.

Serving Methods:

1. Slice and serve over a bed of quinoa for a protein-packed meal.
2. Chop and toss into a vibrant salad for a light lunch.

Turkey and Quinoa Stuffed Peppers

Ingredients:

- 4 bell peppers, halved and seeds removed

- 1 pound ground turkey

- 1 cup cooked quinoa

- 1 cup diced tomatoes

- 1/2 cup black beans, drained and rinsed

- 1 teaspoon cumin

- 1 teaspoon chili powder

- Salt and pepper to taste

Prep Time: 20 minutes

Cooking Time: 25 minutes

Serving Time: 5 minutes

Nutritional Info: (per serving)

- Calories: 250

- Protein: 20g

- Carbohydrates: 25g

- Fat: 8g

- Fiber: 6g

Directions:

- Preheat the oven to 375°F (190°C).

- In a skillet, brown ground turkey.

- Combine turkey, cooked quinoa, diced tomatoes, black beans, cumin, chili powder, salt, and pepper in a bowl.

- Stuff the pepper halves with the mixture and bake for 25 minutes.

- Serve with a dollop of Greek yogurt.

Serving Methods:

1. Top with shredded cheese and broil for a cheesy crust.
2. Pair with a side of roasted sweet potatoes for a well-rounded meal.

Salmon with Dill and Lemon

Ingredients:

- 4 salmon fillets

- 2 tablespoons fresh dill, chopped

- 1 lemon, thinly sliced

- 2 tablespoons olive oil

- Salt and pepper to taste

Prep Time: 10 minutes

Cooking Time: 15 minutes

Serving Time: 5 minutes

Nutritional Info: (per serving)

- Calories: 280
- Protein: 30g
- Carbohydrates: 1g
- Fat: 17g
- Fiber: 0g

Directions: Preheat the oven to 400°F (200°C).

- Place salmon fillets on a baking sheet.
- Season with salt, pepper, and chopped dill.
- Lay lemon slices over each fillet and drizzle with olive oil.
- Bake for 15 minutes or until the salmon flakes easily.
- Serve with a side of steamed asparagus.

Serving Methods:

1. Flake and toss with whole wheat pasta for a hearty dish.
2. Serve over a bed of sautéed spinach for added greens.

Chicken and Vegetable Stir-Fry

Ingredients: 1 pound boneless, skinless chicken breasts, thinly sliced

- 2 cups broccoli florets
- 1 red bell pepper, thinly sliced

- 1 carrot, julienned

- 2 tablespoons soy sauce

- 1 tablespoon hoisin sauce

- 1 tablespoon sesame oil

- 1 teaspoon ginger, minced

- Brown rice for serving

Prep Time: 20 minutes

Cooking Time: 15 minutes

Serving Time: 5 minutes

Nutritional Info: (per serving)

- Calories: 300

- Protein: 28g

- Carbohydrates: 20g

- Fat: 12g

- Fiber: 4g

Directions:

- In a wok or skillet, stir-fry chicken until browned.

- Add broccoli, bell pepper, and carrot, and cook until vegetables are tender-crisp.

- In a small bowl, mix soy sauce, hoisin sauce, sesame oil, and minced ginger.

- Pour the sauce over the chicken and vegetables, stirring to combine.

- Serve over brown rice.

Serving Methods:

1. Wrap in lettuce leaves for a carb-conscious option.
2. Sprinkle with sesame seeds and green onions for added flavor.

Spiced Turkey Burgers

Ingredients:

- 1 pound ground turkey
- 1/2 cup finely chopped red onion
- 1 teaspoon cumin
- 1 teaspoon paprika
- Salt and pepper to taste
- Whole grain buns
- Avocado slices for topping

Prep Time: 15 minutes

Cooking Time: 10 minutes

Serving Time: 5 minutes

Nutritional Info: (per serving)

- Calories: 220
- Protein: 25g
- Carbohydrates: 20g
- Fat: 7g
- Fiber: 3g

Directions:

- In a bowl, mix ground turkey, chopped red onion, cumin, paprika, salt, and pepper.
- Form into burger patties.
- Grill for 4-5 minutes per side or until cooked through.
- Serve on whole grain buns with avocado slices.

Serving Methods:

1. Top with a spicy yogurt sauce for an extra kick.
2. Wrap in lettuce leaves for a low-carb alternative.

Herb-Crusted Baked Chicken Thighs

Ingredients:

- 4 bone-in, skin-on chicken thighs
- 2 tablespoons olive oil
- 1 tablespoon fresh rosemary, chopped
- 1 tablespoon fresh thyme, chopped
- 1 tablespoon fresh parsley, chopped
- 2 cloves garlic, minced
- Salt and pepper to taste

Prep Time: 15 minutes

Cooking Time: 35 minutes

Serving Time: 5 minutes

Nutritional Info: (per serving)

- Calories: 280
- Protein: 25g
- Carbohydrates: 0g
- Fat: 20g
- Fiber: 0g

Directions:

- Preheat the oven to 400°F (200°C).
- Rub chicken thighs with olive oil and season with salt and pepper.
- Mix chopped rosemary, thyme, parsley, and minced garlic.
- Press the herb mixture onto each chicken thigh.
- Bake for 35 minutes or until the skin is crispy.
- Serve with roasted Brussels sprouts.

Serving Methods:

1. Pair with a side of cauliflower mash for a low-carb option.
2. Drizzle with balsamic reduction for added depth of flavor.

Lemon Garlic Shrimp Skewers

Ingredients: 1 pound large shrimp, peeled and deveined

- Zest and juice of 1 lemon
- 2 tablespoons olive oil
- 3 cloves garlic, minced
- 1 teaspoon smoked paprika
- Salt and pepper to taste

Prep Time: 10 minutes

Cooking Time: 5 minutes

Serving Time: 5 minutes

Nutritional Info: (per serving)

- Calories: 160
- Protein: 20g
- Carbohydrates: 2g
- Fat: 8g
- Fiber: 0g

Directions:

- In a bowl, mix lemon zest, lemon juice, olive oil, minced garlic, smoked paprika, salt, and pepper.
- Thread shrimp onto skewers and brush with the lemon garlic mixture.
- Grill for 2-3 minutes per side until shrimp turn pink.
- Serve over a bed of zucchini noodles.

Serving Methods:

1. Toss with whole wheat spaghetti for a complete meal.
2. Squeeze extra lemon juice for a refreshing touch.

Balsamic Glazed Turkey Meatballs

Ingredients: 1 pound ground turkey

- 1/2 cup breadcrumbs (whole wheat or gluten-free)

- 1/4 cup grated Parmesan cheese

- 1 egg

- 2 cloves garlic, minced

- 1/4 cup balsamic glaze

- Fresh basil for garnish

Prep Time: 15 minutes

Cooking Time: 20 minutes

Serving Time: 5 minutes

Nutritional Info: (per serving)

- Calories: 220

- Protein: 20g

- Carbohydrates: 10g

- Fat: 10g

- Fiber: 1g

Directions: Preheat the oven to 375°F (190°C).

- In a bowl, combine ground turkey, breadcrumbs, Parmesan, egg, and minced garlic.

- Form into meatballs and place on a baking sheet.

- Bake for 20 minutes or until cooked through.

- Drizzle with balsamic glaze and garnish with fresh basil.

Serving Methods:

1. Serve over quinoa or brown rice for a wholesome meal.

2. Skewer with toothpicks for a delightful appetizer.

Curry Chicken Lettuce Wraps

Ingredients:

- 1 pound chicken breast, cooked and shredded
- 1 tablespoon curry powder
- 1/2 cup Greek yogurt
- 1/4 cup mango, diced
- 2 tablespoons cilantro, chopped
- Bibb lettuce leaves for wrapping

Prep Time: 15 minutes

Serving Time: 5 minutes

Nutritional Info: (per serving)

- Calories: 230
- Protein: 25g
- Carbohydrates: 8g
- Fat: 10g
- Fiber: 2g

Directions: In a bowl, mix shredded chicken with curry powder.

- Combine with Greek yogurt, diced mango, and chopped cilantro.
- Spoon the mixture onto Bibb lettuce leaves.
- Serve with a side of jicama sticks.

Serving Methods:

1. Top with shredded coconut for a tropical twist.

2. Add a squeeze of lime for extra zing.

Mediterranean Grilled Lamb Chops

Ingredients:

- 8 lamb chops
- 2 tablespoons olive oil
- 1 tablespoon dried oregano
- 1 teaspoon minced garlic
- Zest and juice of 1 lemon
- Salt and pepper to taste

Prep Time: 15 minutes

Cooking Time: 10 minutes

Serving Time: 5 minutes

Nutritional Info: (per serving)

- Calories: 300
- Protein: 30g
- Carbohydrates: 1g
- Fat: 20g
- Fiber: 0g

Directions:

- Preheat the grill to medium-high heat.
- Rub lamb chops with olive oil, dried oregano, minced garlic, lemon zest, salt, and pepper.
- Grill for 4-5 minutes per side for medium-rare.

- Drizzle with lemon juice before serving.
- Serve with a side of Greek salad.

Serving Methods:

1. Pair with couscous for a Mediterranean-inspired dinner.
2. Garnish with crumbled feta cheese for added richness.

Teriyaki Salmon Skewers

Ingredients:

- 1 pound salmon fillets, cut into chunks
- 1/4 cup low-sodium teriyaki sauce
- 2 tablespoons rice vinegar
- 1 tablespoon honey
- 1 teaspoon grated ginger
- Sesame seeds for garnish

Prep Time: 15 minutes

Cooking Time: 10 minutes

Serving Time: 5 minutes

Nutritional Info: (per serving)

- Calories: 250
- Protein: 25g
- Carbohydrates: 10g
- Fat: 12g
- Fiber: 1g

Directions

- In a bowl, whisk together teriyaki sauce, rice vinegar, honey, and grated ginger.
- Marinate salmon chunks in the mixture for 10-15 minutes.
- Thread onto skewers and grill for 5 minutes per side.
- Sprinkle with sesame seeds before serving.
- Serve with a side of steamed broccoli.

Serving Methods:

1. Pair with brown rice for a complete Asian-inspired meal.
2. Serve over a bed of mixed greens for a light lunch.

Baked Turkey Zucchini Boats

Ingredients:

- 4 large zucchini, halved lengthwise
- 1 pound lean ground turkey
- 1 cup tomato sauce
- 1 teaspoon Italian seasoning
- 1/2 cup shredded mozzarella cheese
- Fresh basil for garnish

Prep Time: 20 minutes

Cooking Time: 25 minutes

Serving Time: 5 minutes

Nutritional Info: (per serving)

- Calories: 230
- Protein: 20g
- Carbohydrates: 10g
- Fat: 12g
- Fiber: 3g

Directions: Preheat the oven to 375°F (190°C).

- Scoop out the center of the zucchini halves to create "boats."
- In a skillet, brown ground turkey and season with Italian seasoning.
- Fill each zucchini boat with the turkey mixture.
- Top with tomato sauce and shredded mozzarella.
- Bake for 20-25 minutes until the cheese is melted and bubbly.
- Garnish with fresh basil before serving.

Serving Methods:

1. Serve over quinoa for an added protein boost.
2. Drizzle with balsamic glaze for a flavor enhancement.

Stuffed Bell Peppers with Lean Beef

Ingredients:

- 4 bell peppers, halved and seeds removed
- 1 pound lean ground beef
- 1 cup cooked quinoa
- 1 cup diced tomatoes
- 1/2 cup corn kernels (fresh or frozen)

- 1 teaspoon cumin

- 1 teaspoon chili powder

- Salt and pepper to taste

Prep Time: 25 minutes

Cooking Time: 30 minutes

Serving Time: 5 minutes

Nutritional Info: (per serving)

- Calories: 280

- Protein: 25g

- Carbohydrates: 20g

- Fat: 10g

- Fiber: 4g

Directions:

- Preheat the oven to 375°F (190°C).

- In a skillet, brown ground beef.

- Combine beef with cooked quinoa, diced tomatoes, corn, cumin, chili powder, salt, and pepper.

- Fill each bell pepper half with the mixture.

- Bake for 25-30 minutes until peppers are tender.

- Serve with a dollop of Greek yogurt.

Serving Methods:

1. Top with sliced avocado for a creamy finish.

2. Sprinkle with chopped cilantro for a burst of freshness.

Honey Mustard Glazed Chicken Thighs

Ingredients:

- 4 bone-in, skin-on chicken thighs
- 2 tablespoons Dijon mustard
- 1 tablespoon whole-grain mustard
- 2 tablespoons honey
- 1 tablespoon olive oil
- 1 teaspoon dried thyme
- Salt and pepper to taste

Prep Time: 15 minutes

Cooking Time: 30 minutes

Serving Time: 5 minutes

Nutritional Info: (per serving)

- Calories: 290
- Protein: 24g
- Carbohydrates: 10g
- Fat: 18g
- Fiber: 0g

Directions:

- Preheat the oven to 375°F (190°C).
- In a bowl, whisk together Dijon mustard, whole-grain mustard, honey, olive oil, dried thyme, salt, and pepper.
- Coat chicken thighs with the mustard mixture.

- Bake for 30 minutes or until the skin is golden and crispy.
- Serve with roasted Brussels sprouts.

Serving Methods:

1. Drizzle with extra honey mustard sauce for a sweet kick.
2. Pair with quinoa and steamed green beans for a well-balanced meal.

Mushroom and Spinach Stuffed Chicken Breast

Ingredients:

- 4 boneless, skinless chicken breasts
- 1 cup mushrooms, finely chopped
- 2 cups baby spinach, chopped
- 1/4 cup feta cheese, crumbled
- 2 cloves garlic, minced
- 1 tablespoon olive oil
- Salt and pepper to taste

Prep Time: 20 minutes

Cooking Time: 25 minutes

Serving Time: 5 minutes

Nutritional Info: (per serving)

- Calories: 260
- Protein: 28g

- Carbohydrates: 5g

- Fat: 14g

- Fiber: 2g

Directions:

- Preheat the oven to 400°F (200°C).

- In a skillet, sauté mushrooms, baby spinach, garlic, and olive oil until wilted.

- Butterfly each chicken breast and stuff with the mushroom and spinach mixture.

- Sprinkle with crumbled feta.

- Bake for 25 minutes or until chicken is cooked through.

- Serve with a side of roasted sweet potatoes.

Serving Methods:

1. Drizzle with balsamic reduction for a tangy twist.
2. Garnish with fresh parsley for added color.

Lemon Herb Grilled Chicken Skewers

Ingredients:

- 1.5 pounds boneless, skinless chicken breasts, cut into cubes

- Zest and juice of 2 lemons

- 3 tablespoons olive oil

- 2 teaspoons fresh rosemary, chopped

- 2 teaspoons fresh thyme, chopped

- Salt and pepper to taste

Prep Time: 20 minutes

Cooking Time: 10 minutes

Serving Time: 5 minutes

Nutritional Info: (per serving)

- Calories: 220
- Protein: 25g
- Carbohydrates: 2g
- Fat: 12g
- Fiber: 1g

Directions:

- In a bowl, combine lemon zest, lemon juice, olive oil, chopped rosemary, chopped thyme, salt, and pepper.
- Marinate chicken cubes in the mixture for 15-20 minutes.
- Thread onto skewers and grill for 4-5 minutes per side.
- Serve with a side of quinoa and steamed broccoli.

Serving Methods:

1. Drizzle with extra lemon juice for a zesty flavor.
2. Serve over a bed of arugula for a light and refreshing meal.

Sesame Ginger Beef Stir-Fry

Ingredients:

- 1 pound sirloin steak, thinly sliced
- 2 tablespoons soy sauce

- 1 tablespoon sesame oil

- 1 tablespoon rice vinegar

- 1 tablespoon honey

- 1 tablespoon fresh ginger, minced

- 2 cloves garlic, minced

- Mixed vegetables (bell peppers, broccoli, snap peas)

Prep Time: 20 minutes

Cooking Time: 15 minutes

Serving Time: 5 minutes

Nutritional Info: (per serving)

- Calories: 280

- Protein: 28g

- Carbohydrates: 12g

- Fat: 12g

- Fiber: 3g

Directions:

- In a bowl, mix soy sauce, sesame oil, rice vinegar, honey, minced ginger, and minced garlic.

- Marinate sliced steak in the mixture for 15 minutes.

- In a wok or skillet, stir-fry the beef until browned.

- Add mixed vegetables and continue stir-frying until tender-crisp.

- Serve over brown rice.

Serving Methods:

1. Garnish with sesame seeds for added crunch.

2. Top with sliced green onions for a pop of color.

Cajun Spiced Turkey Breast

Ingredients:

- 1.5 pounds turkey breast

- 2 tablespoons Cajun seasoning

- 1 tablespoon olive oil

- 1 teaspoon smoked paprika

- 1 teaspoon garlic powder

- Salt and pepper to taste

Prep Time: 15 minutes

Cooking Time: 30 minutes

Serving Time: 5 minutes

Nutritional Info: (per serving)

- Calories: 210

- Protein: 30g

- Carbohydrates: 1g

- Fat: 9g

- Fiber: 0g

Directions: Preheat the oven to 375°F (190°C).

- Rub turkey breast with Cajun seasoning, olive oil, smoked paprika, garlic powder, salt, and pepper.
- Roast for 25-30 minutes or until the internal temperature reaches 165°F (74°C).
- Let it rest before slicing.
- Serve with a side of sautéed green beans.

Serving Methods:

- Drizzle with hot sauce for an extra kick.
- Pair with a refreshing cucumber salad.

Mango Habanero Glazed Chicken Drumsticks

Ingredients: 2 pounds chicken drumsticks

- 1 cup mango puree
- 1 habanero pepper, minced (adjust to taste)
- 1/4 cup honey
- 2 tablespoons apple cider vinegar
- 1 teaspoon ground coriander
- Salt and pepper to taste

Prep Time: 20 minutes

Cooking Time: 40 minutes

Serving Time: 5 minutes

Nutritional Info: (per serving)

- Calories: 250
- Protein: 25g

- Carbohydrates: 20g

- Fat: 8g

- Fiber: 1g

Directions:

- Preheat the oven to 400°F (200°C).

- In a saucepan, combine mango puree, minced habanero, honey, apple cider vinegar, ground coriander, salt, and pepper.

- Simmer over medium heat until the sauce thickens.

- Brush chicken drumsticks with the glaze.

- Bake for 35-40 minutes or until cooked through.

- Serve with a side of quinoa and grilled asparagus.

Serving Methods:

1. Garnish with chopped cilantro for freshness.
2. Pair with a cooling cucumber salsa.

Chimichurri Grilled Steak

Ingredients: 1.5 pounds flank steak

- 1 cup fresh parsley, chopped

- 1/2 cup fresh cilantro, chopped

- 4 cloves garlic, minced

- 1/4 cup red wine vinegar

- 1/2 cup olive oil

- 1 teaspoon crushed red pepper flakes

- Salt and pepper to taste

Prep Time: 25 minutes

Cooking Time: 10 minutes

Serving Time: 5 minutes

Nutritional Info: (per serving)

- Calories: 300
- Protein: 25g
- Carbohydrates: 2g
- Fat: 20g
- Fiber: 1g

Directions: In a food processor, combine chopped parsley, chopped cilantro, minced garlic, red wine vinegar, olive oil, crushed red pepper flakes, salt, and pepper.

- Marinate flank steak in half of the chimichurri sauce for 20 minutes.
- Grill steak for 4-5 minutes per side or to desired doneness.
- Let it rest before slicing.
- Serve with the remaining chimichurri sauce on the side.
- Pair with a side of roasted sweet potatoes.

Serving Methods:

1. Drizzle with extra virgin olive oil for added richness.
2. Top with crumbled feta for a Mediterranean twist.

SOUP RECIPES

Quinoa and Vegetable Soup

Ingredients:

- 1 cup quinoa, rinsed
- 4 cups vegetable broth
- 1 onion, diced
- 2 carrots, chopped
- 2 celery stalks, sliced
- 1 zucchini, diced
- 1 can diced tomatoes
- 1 teaspoon dried thyme
- Salt and pepper to taste

Prep Time: 15 minutes

Cooking Time: 30 minutes

Serving Time: 5 minutes

Nutritional Info: (per serving)

- Calories: 180
- Protein: 6g
- Carbohydrates: 30g
- Fat: 3g
- Fiber: 6g

Directions:

- In a pot, sauté onions, carrots, and celery until softened.
- Add quinoa, vegetable broth, diced tomatoes, zucchini, thyme, salt, and pepper.
- Bring to a boil, then reduce heat and simmer for 20-25 minutes.
- Serve with a sprinkle of fresh parsley.

Serving Methods:

1. Pair with a slice of whole-grain bread for a hearty meal.
2. Top with a dollop of Greek yogurt for added creaminess.

Lentil and Spinach Soup

Ingredients:

- 1 cup dried lentils, rinsed
- 6 cups vegetable broth
- 1 onion, finely chopped
- 2 carrots, diced
- 2 cloves garlic, minced
- 2 cups fresh spinach
- 1 teaspoon cumin
- 1/2 teaspoon smoked paprika
- Salt and pepper to taste

Prep Time: 20 minutes

Cooking Time: 40 minutes

Serving Time: 5 minutes

Nutritional Info: (per serving)

- Calories: 220
- Protein: 15g
- Carbohydrates: 40g
- Fat: 1g
- Fiber: 12g

Directions: In a large pot, sauté onions, carrots, and garlic until softened.

- Add lentils, vegetable broth, cumin, smoked paprika, salt, and pepper.
- Simmer for 30-35 minutes until lentils are tender.

- Stir in fresh spinach and cook until wilted.
- Serve with a squeeze of lemon juice.

Serving Methods:

1. Garnish with a swirl of balsamic reduction for added flavor.
2. Serve with a side of whole-grain crackers for crunch.

Chicken and Vegetable Quinoa Soup

Ingredients:

- 1 cup cooked quinoa
- 4 cups chicken broth
- 1 chicken breast, cooked and shredded
- 1 onion, diced
- 2 carrots, sliced
- 1 cup broccoli florets
- 2 cloves garlic, minced
- 1 teaspoon dried thyme
- Salt and pepper to taste

Prep Time: 15 minutes

Cooking Time: 25 minutes

Serving Time: 5 minutes

Nutritional Info: (per serving)

- Calories: 230
- Protein: 20g
- Carbohydrates: 30g
- Fat: 3g
- Fiber: 5g

Directions:

- In a pot, sauté onions and garlic until translucent.

- Add chicken broth, cooked quinoa, shredded chicken, carrots, broccoli, thyme, salt, and pepper.
- Simmer for 15-20 minutes until vegetables are tender.
- Adjust seasoning as needed.
- Serve with a sprinkle of chopped parsley.

Serving Methods:

1. Top with a spoonful of plain yogurt for a creamy texture.
2. Pair with a side of mixed greens for a light lunch.

Tomato Basil Soup with White Beans

Ingredients:

- 2 cans diced tomatoes
- 4 cups vegetable broth
- 1 onion, chopped
- 2 cloves garlic, minced
- 1 can white beans, drained and rinsed
- 1/4 cup fresh basil, chopped
- 1 teaspoon dried oregano
- Salt and pepper to taste

Prep Time: 15 minutes

Cooking Time: 25 minutes

Serving Time: 5 minutes

Nutritional Info: (per serving)

- Calories: 160
- Protein: 7g
- Carbohydrates: 30g
- Fat: 1g
- Fiber: 7g

Directions:

- In a pot, sauté onions and garlic until fragrant.
- Add diced tomatoes, vegetable broth, white beans, basil, oregano, salt, and pepper.
- Simmer for 20 minutes.
- Use an immersion blender to blend until smooth.
- Serve with a drizzle of olive oil.

Serving Methods:

1. Pair with a grilled cheese sandwich for a classic combination.
2. Garnish with a sprinkle of Parmesan cheese for extra richness.

Spicy Kale and Chickpea Soup

Ingredients:

- 1 bunch kale, stems removed and leaves chopped
- 2 cans chickpeas, drained and rinsed
- 4 cups vegetable broth
- 1 onion, finely chopped
- 2 carrots, diced
- 2 teaspoons curry powder
- 1/2 teaspoon cayenne pepper
- Salt and pepper to taste

Prep Time: 20 minutes

Cooking Time: 30 minutes

Serving Time: 5 minutes

Nutritional Info: (per serving)

- Calories: 200
- Protein: 10g
- Carbohydrates: 35g

- Fat: 2g
- Fiber: 12g

Directions:

- In a pot, sauté onions and carrots until softened.
- Add vegetable broth, chopped kale, chickpeas, curry powder, cayenne pepper, salt, and pepper.
- Simmer for 25-30 minutes until kale is tender.
- Adjust seasoning as needed.
- Serve with a squeeze of lemon juice.

Serving Methods:

1. Top with a dollop of Greek yogurt for creaminess.
2. Pair with a slice of whole-grain bread for a complete meal.

Butternut Squash and Apple Soup

Ingredients:

- 1 butternut squash, peeled and diced
- 2 apples, cored and chopped
- 1 onion, diced
- 4 cups vegetable broth
- 1 teaspoon ground cinnamon
- 1/2 teaspoon nutmeg
- Salt and pepper to taste

Prep Time: 20 minutes

Cooking Time: 30 minutes

Serving Time: 5 minutes

Nutritional Info: (per serving)

- Calories: 180
- Protein: 2g

- Carbohydrates: 45g
- Fat: 1g
- Fiber: 8g

Directions:

- In a pot, sauté onions until translucent.
- Add butternut squash, apples, vegetable broth, cinnamon, nutmeg, salt, and pepper.
- Simmer for 25-30 minutes until squash is tender.
- Use an immersion blender to blend until smooth.
- Serve with a sprinkle of chopped fresh parsley.

Serving Methods:

1. Drizzle with a touch of honey for sweetness.
2. Top with a dollop of plain Greek yogurt for creaminess.

Turmeric Ginger Carrot Soup

Ingredients:

- 1 pound carrots, peeled and chopped
- 1 onion, chopped
- 2 cloves garlic, minced
- 1 tablespoon fresh ginger, grated
- 4 cups vegetable broth
- 1 teaspoon ground turmeric
- 1/2 teaspoon cumin
- Salt and pepper to taste

Prep Time: 15 minutes

Cooking Time: 25 minutes

Serving Time: 5 minutes

Nutritional Info: (per serving)

- Calories: 150
- Protein: 2g
- Carbohydrates: 35g
- Fat: 1g
- Fiber: 8g

Directions:

- In a pot, sauté onions, garlic, and ginger until fragrant.
- Add chopped carrots, vegetable broth, turmeric, cumin, salt, and pepper.
- Simmer for 20 minutes until carrots are tender.
- Use a blender to puree until smooth.
- Serve with a swirl of coconut milk.

Serving Methods:

1. Garnish with chopped cilantro for a burst of freshness.
2. Top with roasted pumpkin seeds for added crunch.

Miso Mushroom Soup

Ingredients:

- 6 cups mushroom broth
- 1 cup shiitake mushrooms, sliced
- 1 cup button mushrooms, sliced
- 3 tablespoons white miso paste
- 2 green onions, sliced
- 1 tablespoon soy sauce
- 1 teaspoon sesame oil

Prep Time: 15 minutes

Cooking Time: 20 minutes

Serving Time: 5 minutes

__Nutritional Info:__ (per serving)

- Calories: 120
- Protein: 5g
- Carbohydrates: 15g
- Fat: 5g
- Fiber: 3g

Directions:

- In a pot, bring mushroom broth to a simmer.
- Add shiitake and button mushrooms, white miso paste, soy sauce, and sesame oil.
- Simmer for 15-20 minutes until mushrooms are tender.
- Adjust seasoning as needed.
- Serve with a sprinkle of sliced green onions.

Serving Methods:

1. Add cooked soba noodles for a heartier version.
2. Top with a poached egg for extra protein.

Roasted Red Pepper and Lentil Soup

Ingredients:

- 1 cup red lentils, rinsed
- 4 cups vegetable broth
- 2 red bell peppers, roasted and chopped
- 1 onion, diced
- 2 cloves garlic, minced
- 1 teaspoon cumin
- 1/2 teaspoon smoked paprika
- Salt and pepper to taste

__Prep Time:__ 20 minutes

__Cooking Time:__ 30 minutes

Serving Time: 5 minutes

Nutritional Info: (per serving)

- Calories: 200
- Protein: 10g
- Carbohydrates: 35g
- Fat: 1g
- Fiber: 10g

Directions:

- In a pot, sauté onions and garlic until softened.
- Add vegetable broth, red lentils, roasted red peppers, cumin, smoked paprika, salt, and pepper.
- Simmer for 25-30 minutes until lentils are cooked.
- Use an immersion blender to puree until smooth.
- Serve with a drizzle of olive oil.

Serving Methods:

1. Top with crumbled feta for a creamy texture.
2. Garnish with a sprinkle of fresh basil for a burst of flavor.

Coconut Curry Cauliflower Soup

Ingredients:

- 1 head cauliflower, chopped
- 1 onion, chopped
- 2 cloves garlic, minced
- 1 can coconut milk
- 4 cups vegetable broth
- 2 tablespoons curry powder
- 1 teaspoon turmeric
- Salt and pepper to taste

Prep Time: 15 minutes

Cooking Time: 25 minutes

Serving Time: 5 minutes

Nutritional Info: (per serving)

- Calories: 180
- Protein: 5g
- Carbohydrates: 25g
- Fat: 8g
- Fiber: 7g

Directions:

- In a pot, sauté onions and garlic until fragrant.
- Add chopped cauliflower, vegetable broth, coconut milk, curry powder, turmeric, salt, and pepper.
- Simmer for 20-25 minutes until cauliflower is tender.
- Use an immersion blender to puree until creamy.
- Serve with a swirl of coconut cream.

Serving Methods:

1. Garnish with toasted coconut flakes for added texture.
2. Pair with quinoa for a complete and satisfying meal.

Spinach and White Bean Soup

Ingredients:

- 2 cans white beans, drained and rinsed
- 6 cups vegetable broth
- 4 cups fresh spinach, chopped
- 1 onion, diced
- 2 carrots, sliced
- 2 cloves garlic, minced
- 1 teaspoon dried rosemary
- Salt and pepper to taste

Prep Time: 15 minutes

Cooking Time: 25 minutes

Serving Time: 5 minutes

Nutritional Info: (per serving)

- Calories: 180
- Protein: 10g
- Carbohydrates: 30g
- Fat: 1g
- Fiber: 8g

Directions:

- In a pot, sauté onions and garlic until softened.
- Add vegetable broth, white beans, chopped spinach, carrots, dried rosemary, salt, and pepper.
- Simmer for 20-25 minutes until vegetables are tender.
- Adjust seasoning as needed.
- Serve with a sprinkle of grated Parmesan.

Serving Methods:

1. Drizzle with extra virgin olive oil for added richness.
2. Top with a squeeze of lemon juice for brightness.

Broccoli and Cheddar Soup

Ingredients:

- 4 cups broccoli florets
- 1 onion, chopped
- 2 cloves garlic, minced
- 4 cups vegetable broth
- 1 cup shredded sharp cheddar cheese

- 1 cup milk (or plant-based milk)
- 2 tablespoons flour
- Salt and pepper to taste

Prep Time: 20 minutes

Cooking Time: 25 minutes

Serving Time: 5 minutes

Nutritional Info: (per serving)

- Calories: 220
- Protein: 12g
- Carbohydrates: 20g
- Fat: 10g
- Fiber: 5g

Directions:

- In a pot, sauté onions and garlic until fragrant.
- Add vegetable broth, broccoli, and bring to a boil. Simmer until broccoli is tender.
- In a separate bowl, whisk flour into milk until smooth. Add to the soup and stir.
- Add shredded cheddar cheese, stirring until melted.
- Season with salt and pepper.
- Serve with a garnish of chopped chives.

Serving Methods:

1. Top with a dollop of Greek yogurt for creaminess.
2. Serve in a bread bowl for a cozy presentation.

Sweet Potato and Black Bean Chili

Ingredients:

- 2 large sweet potatoes, diced

- 2 cans black beans, drained and rinsed
- 1 onion, diced
- 3 cloves garlic, minced
- 1 can diced tomatoes
- 4 cups vegetable broth
- 2 teaspoons chili powder
- 1 teaspoon cumin
- Salt and pepper to taste

Prep Time: 20 minutes

Cooking Time: 30 minutes

Serving Time: 5 minutes

Nutritional Info: (per serving)

- Calories: 240
- Protein: 10g
- Carbohydrates: 45g
- Fat: 1g
- Fiber: 10g

Directions:

- In a pot, sauté onions and garlic until softened.
- Add sweet potatoes, black beans, diced tomatoes, vegetable broth, chili powder, cumin, salt, and pepper.
- Simmer for 25-30 minutes until sweet potatoes are tender.
- Adjust seasoning as needed.
- Serve with a dollop of avocado salsa.

Serving Methods:

1. Top with a sprinkle of shredded Monterey Jack cheese.
2. Pair with a slice of cornbread for a complete meal.

Cabbage and White Bean Detox Soup

Ingredients:

- 1 small cabbage, shredded
- 2 cans white beans, drained and rinsed
- 1 onion, chopped
- 2 carrots, sliced
- 4 cups vegetable broth
- 1 teaspoon turmeric
- 1/2 teaspoon cayenne pepper
- Salt and pepper to taste

Prep Time: 15 minutes

Cooking Time: 25 minutes

Serving Time: 5 minutes

Nutritional Info: (per serving)

- Calories: 160
- Protein: 8g
- Carbohydrates: 30g
- Fat: 1g
- Fiber: 10g

Directions:

- In a pot, sauté onions until translucent.
- Add shredded cabbage, sliced carrots, white beans, vegetable broth, turmeric, cayenne pepper, salt, and pepper.
- Simmer for 20-25 minutes until vegetables are tender.
- Adjust seasoning as needed.
- Serve with a squeeze of lemon juice.

Serving Methods:

- Drizzle with extra virgin olive oil for added richness.
- Top with a dollop of plain Greek yogurt for creaminess.

Tomato Basil and Quinoa Soup

Ingredients:

- 1 cup cooked quinoa
- 4 cups vegetable broth
- 1 can crushed tomatoes
- 1 onion, chopped
- 2 cloves garlic, minced
- 1/4 cup fresh basil, chopped
- 1 teaspoon dried oregano
- Salt and pepper to taste

Prep Time: 15 minutes

Cooking Time: 25 minutes

Serving Time: 5 minutes

Nutritional Info: (per serving)

- Calories: 180
- Protein: 5g
- Carbohydrates: 35g
- Fat: 2g
- Fiber: 6g

Directions:

- In a pot, sauté onions and garlic until fragrant.
- Add vegetable broth, crushed tomatoes, cooked quinoa, fresh basil, dried oregano, salt, and pepper.
- Simmer for 20-25 minutes.
- Adjust seasoning as needed.
- Serve with a sprinkle of grated Parmesan.

Serving Methods:

1. Top with croutons for added crunch.
2. Drizzle with balsamic glaze for a burst of flavor.

Wild Rice and Mushroom Soup

Ingredients:

- 1 cup wild rice, cooked
- 6 cups vegetable broth
- 2 cups mushrooms, sliced
- 1 onion, diced
- 3 cloves garlic, minced
- 1 teaspoon thyme
- 1/2 cup almond milk (or any plant-based milk)
- Salt and pepper to taste

Prep Time: 15 minutes

Cooking Time: 30 minutes

Serving Time: 5 minutes

Nutritional Info: (per serving)

- Calories: 200
- Protein: 7g
- Carbohydrates: 35g
- Fat: 3g
- Fiber: 6g

Directions:

- In a pot, sauté onions and garlic until softened.
- Add mushrooms, thyme, and cook until mushrooms release their moisture.
- Pour in vegetable broth and bring to a simmer.

- Add cooked wild rice and almond milk.
- Season with salt and pepper.
- Simmer for an additional 15-20 minutes.
- Serve with a sprinkle of chopped parsley.

Serving Methods:

1. Garnish with a drizzle of truffle oil for an indulgent touch.
2. Top with toasted sliced almonds for added crunch.

Mexican Black Bean Soup

Ingredients:

- 2 cans black beans, drained and rinsed
- 1 can diced tomatoes with green chilies
- 1 onion, chopped
- 2 cloves garlic, minced
- 1 teaspoon cumin
- 1/2 teaspoon smoked paprika
- 4 cups vegetable broth
- Juice of 1 lime
- Salt and pepper to taste

Prep Time: 15 minutes

Cooking Time: 25 minutes

Serving Time: 5 minutes

Nutritional Info: (per serving)

- Calories: 220
- Protein: 10g
- Carbohydrates: 40g
- Fat: 1g
- Fiber: 12g

Directions:

- In a pot, sauté onions and garlic until fragrant.
- Add black beans, diced tomatoes with green chilies, cumin, smoked paprika, and vegetable broth.
- Simmer for 20-25 minutes.
- Stir in lime juice.
- Season with salt and pepper.
- Serve with a dollop of Greek yogurt.

Serving Methods:

- Garnish with sliced jalapeños for extra heat.
- Top with chopped cilantro for freshness.

Italian Wedding Soup

Ingredients:

- 1/2 pound lean ground turkey
- 1/2 cup breadcrumbs
- 1 egg
- 2 tablespoons grated Parmesan cheese
- 1 onion, finely chopped
- 2 carrots, sliced
- 2 cups spinach, chopped
- 4 cups chicken broth
- 1/2 cup small pasta (acini de pepe or orzo)
- Salt and pepper to taste

Prep Time: 20 minutes

Cooking Time: 30 minutes

Serving Time: 5 minutes

Nutritional Info: (per serving)

- Calories: 250
- Protein: 15g
- Carbohydrates: 25g
- Fat: 10g
- Fiber: 4g

Directions:

- In a bowl, mix ground turkey, breadcrumbs, egg, and Parmesan. Shape into small meatballs.
- In a pot, sauté onions until translucent.
- Add carrots, chicken broth, and bring to a simmer.
- Add pasta and meatballs, cooking until pasta is al dente and meatballs are cooked through.
- Stir in chopped spinach.
- Season with salt and pepper.
- Serve with a sprinkle of fresh basil.

Serving Methods:

1. Top with a drizzle of extra virgin olive oil.
2. Garnish with additional grated Parmesan for richness.

Asian-Inspired Tofu Noodle Soup

Ingredients:

- 8 oz firm tofu, cubed
- 4 oz rice noodles
- 4 cups vegetable broth
- 1 tablespoon soy sauce
- 1 teaspoon sesame oil
- 1 cup bok choy, chopped
- 2 green onions, sliced
- 1 tablespoon fresh ginger, grated
- 1 clove garlic, minced

Prep Time: 15 minutes

Cooking Time: 20 minutes

Serving Time: 5 minutes

Nutritional Info: (per serving)

- Calories: 220
- Protein: 12g
- Carbohydrates: 30g
- Fat: 5g
- Fiber: 3g

Directions:

- In a pot, sauté ginger and garlic until fragrant.
- Add vegetable broth, soy sauce, and sesame oil. Bring to a simmer.
- Add rice noodles and cook until tender.
- Stir in cubed tofu and bok choy, cooking until tofu is heated through and bok choy is wilted.
- Season with salt and pepper.
- Serve with a sprinkle of sliced green onions.

Serving Methods:

1. Top with a dash of sriracha for a spicy kick.
2. Garnish with a few cilantro leaves for freshness.

Creamy Asparagus and Potato Soup

Ingredients:

- 1 bunch asparagus, trimmed and chopped
- 2 potatoes, peeled and diced
- 1 onion, chopped
- 2 cloves garlic, minced
- 4 cups vegetable broth

- 1/2 cup plain Greek yogurt
- 1 tablespoon olive oil
- Salt and pepper to taste

Prep Time: 20 minutes

Cooking Time: 30 minutes

Serving Time: 5 minutes

Nutritional Info: (per serving)

- Calories: 180
- Protein: 8g
- Carbohydrates: 30g
- Fat: 5g
- Fiber: 6g

Directions:

- In a pot, sauté onions and garlic until softened.
- Add vegetable broth, chopped asparagus, diced potatoes, and bring to a simmer.
- Cook until vegetables are tender.
- Use an immersion blender to puree until smooth.
- Stir in Greek yogurt, olive oil, salt, and pepper.
- Serve with a garnish of chopped chives.

Serving Methods:

1. Drizzle with a swirl of truffle-infused oil.
2. Top with a sprinkle of grated Parmesan cheese.

28 DAY MEAL PLAN

DAY 1:

- *Breakfast:* Quinoa and Vegetable Soup

- *Lunch:* Spinach and White Bean Soup

- *Dinner:* Coconut Curry Cauliflower Soup

Day 2:

- *Breakfast:* Sweet Potato and Black Bean Chili

- *Lunch:* Broccoli and Cheddar Soup

- *Dinner:* Tomato Basil and Quinoa Soup

Day 3:

- *Breakfast:* Wild Rice and Mushroom Soup

- *Lunch:* Cabbage and White Bean Detox Soup

- *Dinner:* Creamy Asparagus and Potato Soup

Day 4:

- *Breakfast:* Mexican Black Bean Soup

- *Lunch:* Italian Wedding Soup

- *Dinner:* Asian-Inspired Tofu Noodle Soup

Day 5:

- *Breakfast:* Tomato Basil Soup with White Beans

- *Lunch:* Spicy Kale and Chickpea Soup

- *Dinner:* Miso Mushroom Soup

Day 6:

- *Breakfast:* Chicken and Vegetable Quinoa Soup

- *Lunch:* Butternut Squash and Apple Soup

- *Dinner:* Lentil and Spinach Soup

Day 7:

- *Breakfast:* Roasted Red Pepper and Lentil Soup

- *Lunch:* Turmeric Ginger Carrot Soup

- *Dinner:* Quinoa and Vegetable Soup

Day 8:

- *Breakfast:* Quinoa and Vegetable Soup

- *Lunch:* Spinach and White Bean Soup

- *Dinner:* Coconut Curry Cauliflower Soup

Day 9:

- *Breakfast:* Sweet Potato and Black Bean Chili

- *Lunch:* Broccoli and Cheddar Soup

- *Dinner:* Tomato Basil and Quinoa Soup

Day 10:

- *Breakfast:* Wild Rice and Mushroom Soup

- *Lunch:* Cabbage and White Bean Detox Soup

- *Dinner:* Creamy Asparagus and Potato Soup

Day 11:

- *Breakfast:* Mexican Black Bean Soup
- *Lunch:* Italian Wedding Soup
- *Dinner:* Asian-Inspired Tofu Noodle Soup

Day 12:

- *Breakfast:* Tomato Basil Soup with White Beans
- *Lunch:* Spicy Kale and Chickpea Soup
- *Dinner:* Miso Mushroom Soup

Day 13:

- *Breakfast:* Chicken and Vegetable Quinoa Soup
- *Lunch:* Butternut Squash and Apple Soup
- *Dinner:* Lentil and Spinach Soup

Day 14:

- *Breakfast:* Roasted Red Pepper and Lentil Soup
- *Lunch:* Turmeric Ginger Carrot Soup
- *Dinner:* Quinoa and Vegetable Soup

Day 15:

- *Breakfast:* Quinoa and Vegetable Soup
- *Lunch:* Spinach and White Bean Soup
- *Dinner:* Coconut Curry Cauliflower Soup

Day 16:

- ***Breakfast:*** Sweet Potato and Black Bean Chili

- ***Lunch:*** Broccoli and Cheddar Soup

- ***Dinner:*** Tomato Basil and Quinoa Soup

Day 17:

- ***Breakfast:*** Wild Rice and Mushroom Soup

- ***Lunch:*** Cabbage and White Bean Detox Soup

- ***Dinner:*** Creamy Asparagus and Potato Soup

Day 18:

- ***Breakfast:*** Mexican Black Bean Soup

- ***Lunch:*** Italian Wedding Soup

- ***Dinner:*** Asian-Inspired Tofu Noodle Soup

Day 19:

- ***Breakfast:*** Tomato Basil Soup with White Beans

- ***Lunch:*** Spicy Kale and Chickpea Soup

- ***Dinner:*** Miso Mushroom Soup

Day 20:

- ***Breakfast:*** Chicken and Vegetable Quinoa Soup

- ***Lunch:*** Butternut Squash and Apple Soup

- ***Dinner:*** Lentil and Spinach Soup

Day 21:

- *Breakfast:* Roasted Red Pepper and Lentil Soup

- *Lunch:* Turmeric Ginger Carrot Soup

- *Dinner:* Quinoa and Vegetable Soup

Day 22:

- *Breakfast:* Quinoa and Vegetable Soup

- *Lunch:* Spinach and White Bean Soup

- *Dinner:* Coconut Curry Cauliflower Soup

Day 23:

- *Breakfast:* Sweet Potato and Black Bean Chili

- *Lunch:* Broccoli and Cheddar Soup

- *Dinner:* Tomato Basil and Quinoa Soup

Day 24:

- *Breakfast:* Wild Rice and Mushroom Soup

- *Lunch:* Cabbage and White Bean Detox Soup

- *Dinner:* Creamy Asparagus and Potato Soup

Day 25:

- *Breakfast:* Mexican Black Bean Soup

- *Lunch:* Italian Wedding Soup

- *Dinner:* Asian-Inspired Tofu Noodle Soup

Day 26:

- ***Breakfast:*** Tomato Basil Soup with White Beans

- ***Lunch:*** Spicy Kale and Chickpea Soup

- ***Dinner:*** Miso Mushroom Soup

Day 27:

- ***Breakfast:*** Chicken and Vegetable Quinoa Soup

- ***Lunch:*** Butternut Squash and Apple Soup

- ***Dinner:*** Lentil and Spinach Soup

Day 28:

- ***Breakfast:*** Roasted Red Pepper and Lentil Soup

- ***Lunch:*** Turmeric Ginger Carrot Soup

- ***Dinner:*** Quinoa and Vegetable Soup

CONCLUSION

In conclusion, the "Metabolic Reset Diet Cookbook for Women Over 50" is designed to provide a holistic approach to health and well-being for women in this age group. Understanding metabolism is a foundational element, shedding light on the intricate processes that influence weight management, energy levels, and overall health.

The importance of a metabolic reset for women over 50 cannot be overstated. As the body undergoes natural changes with age, adopting a tailored approach to nutrition and lifestyle becomes crucial. The Metabolic Reset Diet offers a strategic and science-backed solution, emphasizing key principles that contribute to a balanced and rejuvenated metabolism.

The Metabolic Reset Diet is comprehensively explored in the book, delving into its definition, principles, and the science behind its effectiveness. It aims to demystify the diet, making it accessible and practical for women over 50. The inclusion of quick and easy recipes, weekly meal plans, and guidance on incorporating exercise further enhances the adaptability of this diet to individual needs and preferences.

The benefits for women over 50 are multifaceted, addressing not only weight management but also promoting overall health and vitality. From supporting hormonal balance to enhancing energy levels and mental clarity, the Metabolic Reset Diet stands as a valuable resource for women navigating the unique challenges and opportunities that come with aging.

The 28-day meal plan provides a diverse and delicious array of recipes, ensuring a nourishing and enjoyable experience for those following the Metabolic Reset Diet. Whether it's breakfast delights, satisfying dinners, or wholesome soups, the recipes cater to varied tastes while aligning with the principles of the diet.